Telemedicine and Telehealth

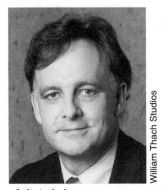

Adam William Darkins, MD, MPH, FRCS, trained as a neurosurgeon in Britain. His clinical background gives him a detailed understanding of the clinical process and the practical difficulties of delivering specialist health care services. During 4 years spent as the medical director at Riverside Community Health Care in London, he implemented telehealth services in the context of contracting to transfer health care services from secondary and tertiary care into primary care. This work directly led to his later use of patient-based clinical information systems to support the brokering of telehealth transactions. He served as a founding member on the board of a national medical directors' organization and worked on major areas of clinical-change management that affect new health care developments. These clinical, organizational-change, and business-development skills underpin his capacity to implement successful telehealth programs. He has written and spoken extensively on telehealth and how it fits with future visions of health care delivery systems that are equitable and sustainable. He helped found the Royal Society of Medicine's Telemedicine Forum and cofounded Global Telemed Ltd. This Northern Ireland-based telehealth company gave him his expertise in defining the new business models on which the future commercial provision of telehealth services are now being based. In addition to his clinical and management experience Adam Darkins has worked directly on patient issues. In the early 1990s he directed a joint project between the King's Fund in London and the Foundation for Informed Medical Decision Making in Hanover, New Hampshire, giving information to patients on treatment choices. He is a past council member of the Patients Association, a national UK patient-advocacy organization. Adam Darkins now lives and works in the United States, where he directs a major telehealth program.

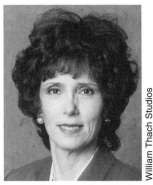

Margaret Ann Cary, MD, MBA, MPH, is a US-trained family physician. Her extensive clinical experience includes practicing in Northern California and Colorado, and directing an emergency room in a remote ski resort. Her extensive knowledge of primary care gives her a familiarity with the challenges of delivering health care far from specialist expertise and of the need to obtain acute health care advice. She moved into medical management after she successfully turned a failing health care facility into a commercial success and her entrepreneurial abilities were recognized. She was an early exponent of the use of telemedicine in primary care situations. Realizing her clinical, managerial, and physician-leadership roles in the state, the Governor of Colorado appointed her to the State Board of Medical Examiners. She served on this Board, the licensing and disciplining agency that regulates physician practice, from 1988 to 1994. This experience gave her firsthand knowledge of the general legal and regulatory framework that underlies the practice of medicine and how this directly impacts the development of telemedicine in the United States. Margaret Cary was actively involved in establishing Denver's World Trade Center at a time when Denver was emerging as a major global center for telecommunications. This work forms the basis for her understanding of the importance of partnerships with telecommunications suppliers in the telephone and cable industries for the future digital delivery of health care services.

Dr. Cary formalized her management education at the University of Colorado where she graduated as the Outstanding MBA Graduate of her year. Subsequently she established a health care communications company with areas of interest that have included physician training, leadership development, and the independent production of health care television programs.

Telemedicine and Telehealth

Principles, Policies, Performance, and Pitfalls

Adam William Darkins, MD, MPH, FRCS
Margaret Ann Cary, MD, MBA, MPH

 Springer Publishing Company

Springer Publishing Company, Inc.
536 Broadway
New York, NY 10012-3955

Acquisitions Editor: Bill Tucker
Production Editor: Pamela Lankas
Cover design by James Scotto-Lavino

01 02 03 04 / 5 4 3

Library of Congress Cataloging-in-Publication-Data

Darkins, Adam William
    Telemedicine and telehealth : principles, policies, performance, and pitfalls / Adam William Darkins and Margaret Ann Cary.
        p. ; cm.
    Includes bibliographical references and index.
    ISBN 0-8261-1302-8 (hardcover)
        1. Telecommunication in medicine.   I. Cary, Margaret Ann.   II. Title.
    [DNLM: 1. Telemedicine—organization & administration. W 83 D219t 2000]
    R119.9 .D37 2000
    362.1—dc21
                                                                            99-050386

Printed in the United States of America

Contents

Introduction

Telecommunications technologies are changing ways of thinking, acting, and communicating throughout the world. The new age dawning has a title, *the Information Age*. What does the Information Age mean for us, and how will our lives change in the future as a result? There are no clear answers to these questions yet. A complex interaction of social, cultural, economic, and technical factors, with large measures of serendipity thrown in, will decide these aspects of our future. Telemedicine and telehealth form just one part of a vast virtual jigsaw puzzle assembling before our eyes—a jigsaw puzzle in which ever more of us participate as the World Wide Web grows and digital data networks proliferate.

In this book on telemedicine and telehealth we explore how the medical, social, cultural, and economic dimensions associated with these digital data networks will affect the kinds of health care services we can expect to receive in the future. Our intention is not to idly theorize in what we write. Instead, we have tried to present a framework for the array of people and professions involved in creating telemedicine and telehealth networks to use in understanding how to work together more effectively. Until comparatively recently, health care used to be the exclusive preserve of the health professions—medicine, nursing, and the professions allied with medicine. Real change began in the 1980s, when general management systems were introduced and a new cadre of general managers entered the health care arena. Since then the health care professions have had to adapt further with the emergence of health care markets and the growth of managed care during the 1990s. A new millennium now looks set to bring yet another culture shock. The Information Age is bringing a new generation of information scientists, together with the hardware and software technologies they generate, into the field of health care. A health care industry largely based on anecdotes, precedents, and conventions now has the challenge of embracing knowledge engineering systems and so provide more appropriate, effective, and cost-effective health care to the population's seemingly insatiable demand for this. Perhaps the greatest dilemma associated with all these changes is how to ensure that innovations in the process of delivering care are not achieved at the expense of sacrificing widely accepted values of what constitutes the humanity of care.

Telehealth involves new, multidisciplinary ways of working and can bring health care directly to patients. If telehealth services are properly introduced and based on "evidence of effectiveness," we believe telehealth has the capacity to improve the *quality* of health care, provide equity of *access* to health care services, and reduce the *cost* of delivering health care. Achieving these goals requires that communication channels develop between the different disciplines involved in delivering telehealth services. This book is intended as a bridge to develop a shared understanding of the key issues among people and professions with different cultural and intellectual perspectives. We attempt to construct this bridge from practical advice on how we believe intersecting processes must be managed if telehealth programs are to work in the eyes of patients and practitioners.

This book is not a linear thinker's guide, trying to give the ten basic rules to making a telehealth project work. We do not view the future development of telehealth in straight-line terms. Processes in the world around us increasingly seem nonlinear. The development of telehealth, with its social, cultural, economic, technical, and ethical dimensions, is exactly the crucible of interactions in which complexity theory rather than linear dynamics operates. In our book we hope to stimulate the passion and energy of people in whatever field or whatever profession they work in to add their contribution of the vital human spark needed to make telehealth happen.

Health care systems around the world all seem to have similarly insoluble equations to solve. Lack of clear answers fits with the complex nature of the global environment in which we now all live and work. The perspectives we bring in writing this book are those of a male British-trained specialist physician who has worked in the British National Health Service and now works in the United States, and of a female U.S. family physician who has trained and worked in the United States and United Kingdom. We have both worked in public health, health management, and health policy development as well as in promoting the emergence of telehealth. We interweave these clinical, public health, management, and policy considerations throughout the book. The impact these considerations have on telemedicine and telehealth are global rather than strictly national. However, a truly global interpretation of telehealth soon becomes very complex because of the variations in the types of health care systems and the changing telecommunications environments in which they operate. We have therefore chosen mainly to contrast the development of telemedicine and telehealth in the U.S. and British health care systems. This offers a backdrop of private versus nationalized health care systems existing in countries with highly competitive and deregulated telecommunications environments. We look at the development of telemedicine and telehealth and assess a range of models and solutions to make telehealth work in different health care situations.

Telehealth is a huge new field of endeavor and one in which many of the waters are uncharted. Uncertainty and challenge coexist with excitement in developing telemedicine and telehealth services. Not only have we many *unknowns* in telemedicine and telehealth, what is *known* changes all the time—new facts are learned and old concepts discounted. We have painted pictures, developed scenarios, and provided information that we believed were true to the best of our knowledge at the time of writing this book. We urge all those taking suggestions and facts from our book to use in developing telehealth services to check on whether these facts and opinions apply in their own situation or country and are still true. We believe telemedicine and telehealth must be based on *evidence of effectiveness.* Those managing new projects must critically develop their own evidence base and not passively rely on old evidence.

In the 21st century the greatest challenge facing health care systems is how to make universal health care coverage available to populations. We could not feed ourselves if we relied on the agrarian systems of the Middle Ages, and yet vast world disparity in access to food remains even so. It seems unlikely that late 20th-century systems of health care delivery in the United States and the United Kingdom can adequately deliver health care coverage for the population, any more than the agrarian systems of the Middle Ages could now provide enough food. If telemedicine and telehealth are going to provide the solutions we need in health care, the main problem is how to fit people to the technology rather than the development of the technology itself. The main reward from telehealth promises to be greater access of people to health care services. Will the problems thwart the promised rewards? Only time and complexity theory can tell. We have no judgments to make on the changes we see happening, only a need to find common solutions that work.

1

Definitions of Telemedicine and Telehealth and a History of the Remote Management of Disease

Many definitions of telemedicine and telehealth are confusing because they try to be all-embracing and in doing so lose touch with the essential elements of what they were originally intended to describe. Newly made-up jargon and obscure technological terms often form the semantic membership badge of a newly emerging discipline. This obstacle is certainly true in telemedicine and telehealth, where it is easy to become entangled in complex descriptions and so feel excluded from it by the technobabble. We have tried to avoid this by using existing definitions of telemedicine and telehealth, definitions that are concise and practical yet fluid enough to keep pace with this rapidly emerging field. We chose not to add to the possible confusion by creating our own new set of definitions, preferring instead to use those of others that we believe capture the current sense of the wide range of health care activity encompassed by telemedicine and telehealth.

We recommend taking a laissez-faire approach to accepting any single definition. This is because we believe that it is more important that the principles underlying telemedicine and telehealth be grasped than cloaked in mystery and set in stone. In the world of information technology constant change is a given. Computer processing power is now doubling in less than 18 months. Applications for technologies constantly evolve, so rigid definitions can become as redundant as yesterday's technology. The particular excitement of working with information technology in health care is about how it makes change happen. Telemedicine and telehealth promise to bring untold change to the health care industry and radically improve the delivery of care to patients. Because of their capacity to revolutionize health care we believe definitions of telemedicine and telehealth should reflect the fundamentals of delivering health care remotely, without academic agonizing about what technical platform is being used.

SHOULD IT BE TELEMEDICINE OR TELEHEALTH?

The word *telemedicine* became prominent in health care in the early 1990s. In the 21st century we foresee telemedicine as it is currently defined extending far beyond delivering medical care, so we prefer the term *telehealth* to telemedicine to describe these wider applications. Some current definitions of telemedicine and telehealth in the literature include the following:

Telemedicine Definition 1

Telemedicine involves the use of modern information technology, especially two-way interactive audio/video communications, computers, and telemetry, to deliver health services to remote patients and to facilitate information exchange between primary care physicians and specialists at some distances from each other.[1]

Telemedicine Definition 2

Telemedicine is health care carried out at a distance.[2]

Telemedicine Definition 3

Telemedicine—the use of advanced telecommunications technologies to exchange health information and provide healthcare services across geographic, time, social and cultural barriers.[3]

Telemedicine Definition 4

The World Health Organization (WHO) makes a distinction between telemedicine and telehealth: *If telehealth is understood to mean the integration of telecommunications systems into the practice of protecting and promoting health, while telemedicine is the incorporation of these systems into curative medicine, then it must be acknowledged that telehealth corresponds more closely to the international activities of WHO in the field of public health. It covers education for health, public and community health, health systems development and epidemiology, whereas telemedicine is orientated more towards the clinical aspect.*[4]

The definitions we quote contain similar elements. We feel it is largely a question of an individual's preference as to which one to adopt. We understand why the WHO's definition makes its distinction between telemedicine and telehealth. However, in the long term we believe this distinction will become unnecessary. Purchasers of health care services are contracting for a continuum of services that extends from health promotion, disease prevention, and curative treatments through to palliative care. Telemedicine can be applied to the complete range of health care interventions and is not and should not be limited to delivering curative medical treatment for established disease. Pragmatically, we think it is much more realistic if telemedicine is thought of as a subset of a wider entity called telehealth. If the narrower concept of telemedicine becomes subsumed into a wider vision of telehealth, then telemedicine becomes an unnecessary term to use. This is the reason that we increasingly see the term telemedicine giving way to telehealth.

We see practical advantages to using telehealth instead of telemedicine as a term to describe remotely delivering health services care. Telemedicine implies that the remote delivery of health care is exclusively associated with physicians. Although physicians are key professionals in health care and must often be directly involved in delivering services by face-to-face contact and telehealth, the physician's role is changing. Physicians are now frequently working as members of wider teams of health care practitioners and less often as autonomous individuals. To use a term that singles out one of the disciplines, whether medicine, nursing, or another, as being of singular importance in the remote delivery of health care fails to acknowledge the importance of an overall team approach to delivering care. As telemedicine has become more involved in newer growth areas, such as delivering home health care services and giving health information to patients and practitioners, we find that health care organizations drop the word *telemedicine* in favor of the more accurate and egalitarian title *telehealth* for their projects.

We feel no blind allegiance to using either word nor to any future replacement for these words. Our primary concern is with the practical consequences of delivering health care in situations where patient and practitioner are remote from one another and where information technology systems provide the bridge for clinical communication. The words should simply be a tool to understand what is occurring. With this in mind it is interesting that the word *telehealth* derives from adding the prefix *tele-* to the word *health;* the word *telemedicine,* from adding the same prefix to the word *medicine. Tele-* comes from an ancient Greek word of the same spelling, meaning "distant."[5] These word derivations suggest working definitions with which we are comfortable. Telemedicine is quite literally medicine practiced at a distance, and telehealth is the delivery of health care services at a distance. These are represented diagrammatically in Figure 1.1.

THE HISTORY OF TELEHEALTH

The current hyperbole surrounding telemedicine/telehealth suggests that it is a revolution in the delivery of health care. Telemedicine/telehealth is frequently associated in definitions and in people's minds with using television, computers, radio, the Internet, videotapes, and fax machines. This association is understandable because these are now the communications media we commonly use, and they are what make telehealth as many currently conceive it to be possible. A definition of telehealth as synonymous with current information technology systems misses the fact that as humans we were able to communicate information about states of health over distances long before these modern technologies were available. Simple devices such as bells, flags, and signs were used for this purpose in the past. Improvements in the health of populations, such as our current life expectancies in the United States and the United Kingdom, have resulted more from public health measures introduced to combat infectious disease than from new medical technologies.[6] Before the mid-20th century, infectious disease was the main cause of mortality and morbidity in the United States and Western Europe.[6] Until relatively recently, health care systems were preoccupied with trying to prevent death from major outbreaks of communicable disease. This meant they were much less concerned with the effects of heart disease, diabetes, and stroke. Health care at a distance, or telehealth, has been practiced since antiquity, using primitive communication technologies to prevent and control the spread of infectious disease.

Leprosy has affected large numbers of people throughout human history. It mainly occurs in tropical and subtropical parts of the world. Leprosy still remains a major cause of morbidity and mortality. Long before people understood the cause of leprosy was an infectious agent, *Mycobacterium leprae,* they realized it spread from those affected to those who were not. People with leprosy were avoided and segregated from nonsufferers in an effort to escape contracting the disease. The avoidance devices employed to

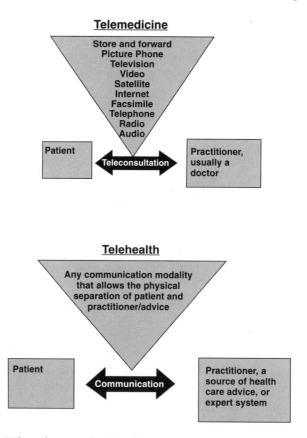

Figure 1.1   Telemedicine and telehealth.

do this included the convention of making lepers ring bells to warn others not to come near.

This is an early example of transmitting health information at a distance. Before it was known bubonic plague spread to humans because of a bite from an oriental rat flea infected with *Pasteurella pestis* and then was passed from person to person, people knew plague failed to spread if those affected were isolated for a period of time. Ships carrying the plague flew yellow flags to indicate their ship was in quarantine and to keep other ships away. When the Great Plague affected the village of Eyam in the north of England, villagers mounted signs and posted lookouts to keep all visitors away until all who were going to die had done so. Through this unselfish action, although most of the village died, the spread of plague into surrounding towns and villages was prevented.

These past attempts at transmitting health information may well seem crude to us now. We have sophisticated technology quite literally at our fingertips. Some purists who equate telemedicine with sophisticated technology would summarily reject the past use of bells and flags to ward off infectious disease as examples of either telemedicine or telehealth. Our reason for including this perspective is not to be pedantic or clever but to suggest there are underlying principles of communication in telehealth that remain the same regardless of the technology used. A unique and distinguishing feature of our being human is an overriding need to communicate words. Exchanging information about our health is a basic ritual of our daily communication with one another. We even include this in our usual daily greetings of "How are you?" and "How do you do?" As new communication technologies come along, we have incorporated these into the ways we communicate about health care and health-related information. However we try to convey information about health care, we are constrained by the limitations our communications technologies impose, our current understanding of disease, and the methods of treatment we have available. The lesson from this for telehealth is how the capacity of any new communications technology to improve our health stems from the power it has to communicate, not from the fine detail of the technology itself.

The first major milestone marking the arrival of telehealth as we now conceive it came with Alexander Graham Bell's invention of the telephone. When his telephone worked for the first time, Bell shouted, "Watson, come here. I need you" into his crude apparatus. Bell was trying to summon help from his assistant, Watson, after sulfuric acid spilled over his hand from an overturned battery.[7] Formal recognition of the role the telephone would play in medicine came later, in 1897, when a telephone was used to diagnose a child with croup and the case was reported in the medical journal *Lancet*.[8] We all recognize the telephone as a ubiquitous tool in society, a tool used in every facet of delivering health care, as shown in Table 1.1.

The start of telemedicine as commonly defined[1,3] dates back to the late 1960s in the United States. This marks the initial use of a closed-circuit television system to provide a routine distance education and teleconsultation facility between the Nebraska Psychiatric Institute and a remote state mental health hospital.[9] In 1965 an early one-time example of telesurgery took place when cardiac surgeon Michael DeBakey performed open heart surgery in the United States and transmitted the procedure live to a hospital in Geneva, Switzerland, using Comsat's Early Bird satellite. Dr DeBakey described the progress of the operation and answered live questions from Geneva.[10]

By 1973 a sufficient mass of early telemedicine activity had been built up throughout the United States to warrant a national conference and workshop on telemedicine in Ann Arbor, Michigan. The content of the conference included discussions about the technical specification of telemedicine

Table 1.1   The Variety of Uses for the Telephone in Health Care

- Summon emergency assistance.
- Get second opinions.
- Schedule health care activities.
- Give remote health care advice.
- Monitor the condition of patients remotely.

systems, the economic and psychological effects of telemedicine, and the scientific evaluation of telemedicine programs.[11] These issues all remain subjects of concern in contemporary telemedicine/telehealth conferences. A highlight of the 1973 conference was the description of how an interactive television project linked Logan International Airport in Boston to the Massachusetts General Hospital.[12] The Logan Airport project showed how real-time video consultation in health care was made possible by using the state-of-the-art technology of the time—black-and-white television cameras and monitors to transmit and receive analog signals.

The wave of enthusiasm for telemedicine in the early 1970s included many of the same promises now being heard in support of telemedicine/telehealth investment such as how it "will make the practice of medicine more efficient and effective." Unfortunately, back in the 1970s these promises could not translate into widespread medical acceptance or continuing financial support for telemedicine. Because telemedicine was unable to create a significant role for itself in the routine practice of health care, one by one the early pilot telemedicine projects folded. In retrospect it seems there were four main reasons this first flowering of telemedicine ended:

1. The high costs of the technology.
2. The poor quality of images.
3. A lack of uptake of services.
4. An inability to interface telemedicine with mainstream health care provision.

A wider political and economic problem contributing to the demise of telemedicine was the general financial climate after the oil crisis of the early 1970s. This global upset curbed the general enthusiasm for high-tech solutions and reduced the funding that governments struggling to cope with the inflationary pressures of increased energy costs could provide.

From the mid-1970s until the mid-1990s the interest of the general health care sector in telemedicine waned. During this fallow period for telemedicine four specialist areas of health care maintained an interest in telemedicine and supported its continued development. These specialist areas of health care are shown in Table 1.2.

Although very different organizations, they all have reasons in common for why they maintained or developed an interest in telemedicine long after it had become unpopular elsewhere as a health care delivery tool. All of the organizations faced a similar dilemma, that of providing medical care to people working in situations that are remote or inaccessible to the usual health care services. Conventional methods of health care delivery could offer either no viable solution or a solution at prohibitive cost. Telemedicine made sense in such situations because it solved problems where the high cost of telemedicine was not an absolute deterrent. Telemedicine development therefore continued in these areas after other health care applications, including many of its early pioneers, abandoned it as impractical and/or too expensive. These telemedicine developments are briefly described below.

The National Aeronautics and Space Agency (NASA) in the United States needed to find ways to monitor the health of astronauts in space. Telehealth was used for research purposes and also to provide remote health care advice in case of an emergency in space.

Antarctic survey stations were (and still are) unable to evacuate sick or injured personnel for several months of the year, when adverse weather conditions and continual darkness make air travel a practical impossibility. Although Antarctic survey stations have resident medical officers, it is logistically impossible to provide sufficient resources of staff and equipment to cover all possible medical emergencies.

Offshore oil exploration rigs regularly face situations where they cannot evacuate sick or injured platform workers by helicopter to get medical care because of weather conditions such as storms. Oil rigs need access to immediate medical advice to treat sick and injured personnel on site or to help support them until evacuation is possible.

The US military has been heavily involved in telemedicine activities around the world. This commitment has developed over the half century from the Second World War to the Bosnian conflict as the US military has faced increasing reluctance of the US public to tolerate casualties in military engagements overseas. The experience of managing the cost and complexity of providing battlefield care for injured soldiers during the Vietnam War prompted the US military to look for other ways of bringing medical expertise closer to those injured in battle, ways involving less risk of injury to health care personnel.[13]

**Table 1.2   Specialist Areas of Telehealth Development
Between 1974 and 1989**

- Health care in space exploration by NASA
- Health care for the various Antarctic surveys
- Health care in the offshore oil exploration industry
- Military health care

The inflationary spirals inspired by the oil crisis started the financial concerns that have beset US and UK health care systems ever since. When inflationary effects hit other sectors of the economy, development projects such as telemedicine in the four types of organizations mentioned above were relatively protected. They were special areas where conventional medical practice could not come up with any obvious alternative apart from telemedicine. Consequently, these telemedicine projects flourished between 1975 and 1989 and faced little of the type of resistance that health care professionals often show when telehealth is introduced into general health care settings. The initial failure of telemedicine in general health care and its later success in specialist situations suggests key variables that determine the success or failure of a telehealth program. These variables are represented in the equation shown in Figure 1.2.

Figure 1.2 suggests the success of a telehealth program directly relates to the quality of its services and their accessibility/acceptability to patients and practitioners in a given health care setting. Consultations from highly qualified practitioners on equipment producing high-quality images enhance the chance of success. If the health care situation chosen for the telehealth service is highly accepting of the service, this will also raise the chance of success. Conversely, the chance of success is inversely proportional to the cost and objections from health care professionals who must use the service or refer to it.

Real interest in using telemedicine to provide health care to the general population was reawakened in Scandinavia during the late 1980s and the early 1990s. The Norwegian government funded 90% of the costs of care in Norway's national health care system. Government social policy in Norway included a commitment to provide universal health care to all its citizens.

$$Telehealth\ Project's\ Success = \frac{Quality\ of\ service\ and\ access\ to\ health\ care\ services}{Cost\ of\ services\ and\ professional\ objection}$$

Figure 1.2   The equation governing the success of a telehealth program.

Equity of access of the population to health care services was an important political issue in Norway. In terms of the success of a telehealth project it was the *quality of service* and *access to health care services* variables from the equation (Figure 1.2) that provided the stimulus for Norway's support of telemedicine programs in the late 1980s. Ironically, it seems as though the oil crisis that played a part in killing off the earlier telemedicine projects both stimulated the Norwegian offshore oil exploration industry and created tax revenues that helped support Norwegian telemedicine activity in the late 1980s.

Norway also had a public health rationale for using telemedicine in the late 1980s and early 1990s. Norway's landmass includes tracts of territory where the population is remote from the amenities of a large city, including specialist health care services. Attracting doctors to provide such services as otolaryngology and pathology in the remote regions of Norway was difficult for two main reasons. First, in such areas of low population density, utilization rates for specialist services can vary widely over time, making such services expensive to provide. Inactivity also frustrates specialist doctors working in remote areas, even if they can be recruited to work there. The second reason is that educational and cultural factors make attracting doctors to work in remote rural areas a problem. After university and postgraduate education, specialist physicians are often loath to leave large cities with their educational and professional links to academic medical centers. Cities also have cultural, social, and gastronomic attractions that are often less available to doctors if they move to and work in remote regions. If it was difficult to physically attract specialists to work in remote parts of Norway, then an alternative solution was to use telemedicine to take the doctors to the patients.

An additional factor in favor of telemedicine was that by the late 1980s telemedicine technology was far more robust and much less expensive than it had been 20 years previously. Particular health care services that were required in the remote areas of Norway were otolaryngology,[14] pathology,[15] and radiology.[16]

So in the early 1990s the primary focus of a renewed wave of interest in telemedicine settled on Norway. The particular health care needs of Norway's remote centers of population favored a telemedicine model based on providing real-time videoconsultation. Real-time videoconsultation enabled a specialist physician at a university hospital to conduct a remote consultation with a general practitioner (GP) and guide the GP through a consultation with a patient by means of a two-way audio and video connection. This made the solution to the specialist physician shortage in remote areas of Norway one of supplying *virtual* specialist physicians. The medical specialties readily adopting teleconsultation included:

- Radiology
- Pathology
- Dermatology
- Psychiatry
- Cardiology
- Otorhinolaryngology

The results of using this videoconsultation model are shown in Table 1.3.

The main reason for the development of telemedicine in Norway during the late 1980s is similar to its development in NASA, the military, Antarctic exploration, and oil exploration. It was used to provide remote care where there seemed no alternative. Because there were no volume producers of telemedicine equipment, the capital costs of these projects were high. In a nationalized health care system costs could be spread over a greater risk pool and justified by the need to provide an equitable service to the population. These projects did not have to take root in the harsh climate of a competitive market for health care services. Reasons for the successful implementation of telemedicine in Norway are suggested in Table 1.4.

The crucial importance of the Norwegian experience of telemedicine in the late 1980s and early 1990s was in showing how telemedicine could effectively deliver routine general health care services. Norwegian telemedicine was government-subsidized, so it could not show whether telemedicine programs would thrive in competitive health care markets. Two other unanswered questions were whether telemedicine had a place in the routine delivery of health care outside remote settings and whether the majority of doctors would support or resist telemedicine in nonremote settings.

During the early 1990s other governments (e.g., UK, New Zealand, and Australia), were preoccupied with the escalating expenses of delivering health care to the general population. All these countries adopted variants of health care markets as mechanisms to contain health care costs. These new market approaches were not fertile environments for the widespread introduction of a new and unproven technology like telemedicine. The governments wanted to know up front who would pay the costs and what were

Table 1.3   The Norwegian Experience of Face-to-Face Teleconsultation in the 1990s[17]

- The diagnostic quality of the teleconsultation equaled conventional face-to-face examinations.
- Patients were able to safely and reliably access the medical expertise they required in their home environment.
- Telemedicine was highly effective and saved the costs of transport.

Table 1.4   Reasons Why Telemedicine Reintroduction Worked in Norway

- A clearly defined clinical need
- Clear financial backing
- An enthusiastic telecommunications partner (Norwegian Telecom)
- The appropriate technology
- Services provided below market cost because of subsidies provided for equipment and by a nationalized health service

the direct benefits of telemedicine over conventional health care delivery. There were no clear data to support telemedicine as an acceptable and cost-effective new model for health care delivery to convince health care systems to buy into it in a big way. Despite these new barriers, the example of telemedicine in Norway reawakened interest in telemedicine worldwide. It spawned new projects in the United Kingdom, the United States, France, Australia, New Zealand, and Hong Kong. However, this second wave of interest in telemedicine has depended heavily on developing niche markets such as prison telemedicine or teleradiology or in attracting grant funding to pump-prime it. The vast majority of telemedicine activity worldwide still remains grant-funded, and right now most could not survive if they relied on selling commercial products to generate revenue to support them in a health care market.

In cost-conscious economic climates, finding a source of outside funding has dictated much of the history of telemedicine during the 1990s. Consequently, telemedicine has been mainly, although by no means exclusively, associated with prison health care and grant-funded rural telemedicine programs. Most telehealth activity now takes place in the United States, although there are notable telemedicine programs in the United Kingdom, New Zealand, Australia, Hong Kong, Canada, and France. In this chapter our brief review of the history of telemedicine concentrates mainly on telemedicine activity in the United States. This is because an overview of the United States experience provides generalizable lessons for programs in other parts of the world. We have not chronicled all the projects in the United States and other countries nor acknowledged key individuals whose personal contributions have made telehealth clinically and organizationally possible. The world of telehealth/telemedicine is a small one, and these individuals and projects are well known. Nonetheless, before we move back to look at the underlying processes affecting the expansion of telehealth, we want to acknowledge the pioneering work of many determined and inspired individuals. Their struggle to bring telehealth projects to life and then through to fruition means we are in a position to seriously access what is happening in telehealth today and consider its future.

In 1995 the main focus of telemedicine activity moved from Scandinavia to the United States when the annual rate of United States telemedicine consultations overtook the number in Norway. The main reasons for the renewed US interest in telemedicine was the promise telemedicine could:

1. provide greater access to health care services for the general population
2. improve the quality of health care services
3. reduce the cost of delivering health care

Because it was sold on the promise of these deliverables explains why the two main growth areas for telemedicine in the United States throughout the 1990s were prison telemedicine and rural telemedicine. These were growth areas because

* In prisons telemedicine promised to save transport costs and improve quality.
* Parts of rural America are as underserved by health care services as were remote parts of Norway.

Prison telemedicine is a rapidly expanding niche market for telemedicine in the United States. One of many notable programs illustrating why this growth has occurred is the Texas prison system program emanating from the University of Texas.[18] The United States prison population is rising by 8%–9% per year, and the prison population has endemic and intractable public health problems.[19] In the Texas prison system inmates have statutory guarantees of access to primary and specialty care services consistent with community standards. Faced with the costs of this entitlement, telemedicine offered the state a possible way to resolve what otherwise seemed an impossible health care delivery equation for Texas. Telemedicine saves transport and security bills for the transfer of prisoners over distances of up to 850 miles from correctional institutions to medical care. State treasuries must bear this overhead of transport and security costs to provide prison health care. Saving these expenses makes more resources available for the direct delivery of services and so increases the efficiency of prison health care. For this reason, prison telemedicine is now seen as an attractive proposition to an increasing number of states.

Rural telemedicine is attractive in the United States because there are parts of the county with similar difficulties in attracting doctors to work as in remote parts of Norway. The situation is illustrated in the state of Georgia, where a statewide telemedicine program was introduced for, among other reasons, a perceived shortage of doctors. In 1992, 11 of Georgia's 159 counties

Table 1.5   The Top Five Reasons for Teleconsultation in the United States During 1996[24]

Specialty for Consultation	Percentage
Mental health	21
Accident and emergency	16
Cardiology	12
Dermatology	11
Surgery	8

had no practicing physicians, and fewer than 50% of counties had a practicing pediatrician.[20] There was a fourfold increase in the numbers of rural telemedicine projects in the United States between 1990 and 1995.[21] The majority of the rural telemedicine programs are either funded by grants or directly from a hospital institution. The most common specialties for teleconsultation in rural areas are radiology, cardiology, and orthopedics, with the majority of rural telemedicine activity limited to teleradiology alone.[22]

Commercial telemedicine activity has grown appreciably in one clinical field in the United States, teleradiology. Recently, the number of diagnostic teleradiology cases read in the United States doubled, from 120,000 per year in 1996 to 250,000 per year in 1997.[23] Some teleradiology providers record their clinical activity rose by as much as 700% between 1996 and 1997. At the end of 1996 there were 80 active telemedicine programs operating in 38 states and Washington, DC.[24] Seventy-two of these programs used real-time interactive videoconsultation (meaning a remote center could get immediate advice from a radiologist). Eight centers used only store-and-forward as the mode of teleconsultation for teleradiology (meaning an image was sent for later reporting by a radiologist elsewhere).

Overall telemedicine activity in the United States is patchy. The main specialties adopting telehealth for teleconsultations using interactive and store-and-forward modes of consultation in the US during 1996 are shown in Table 1.5.

Table 1.6 gives the results of a survey of 72 sites undertaking telemedicine in the United States during 1996. It gives data on the main problems confronting these programs in continuing to provide telehealth services in the future.

At the end of the 1990s big questions hang over the future of the latest flowering of telemedicine. Growth and expansion of telemedicine activity has been mainly supported by grant funding from government or capital investment by hospital providers. Many telemedicine programs exist in

$$\text{Telehealth Project's Success} = \frac{\textit{Quality of service and access to health care service}}{\textit{Cost of services and professional objection}}$$

Figure 1.3   Current areas that impede the success of telehealth.

which the rates of teleconsultation per year are too low for them to have a possible future in any commercial environment. The current challenge for telemedicine programs is to work on the two parts of the telemedicine success equation that have been unsuccessful so far—reducing the costs of delivering care and professional acceptance as shown in Figure 1.3.

We believe a focus on the wider opportunities of telehealth and not just the limited area of telemedicine will fuel the expansion in teleconsultation activity needed to generate the secure revenue streams on which the future of remote health care delivery systems must ultimately depend. The underlying business case to justify a health care organization in making an initial investment in telehealth usually means changing the way in which health care is delivered. Changes in clinical practice are the way in which the cost savings in health care delivery are actually realizable from telemedicine. If introducing telehealth is to achieve these cost savings, invariably, professional practice must change, which can lead to resistance from health care professionals.

We discuss the feasibility of making efficiency gains and changing professional practice elsewhere in this book. However, before considering telehealth's overall future there are valuable lessons to learn from reviewing an existing area of telehealth. This area is already fully accepted in society generally and is fully integrated into all health care delivery systems; it is the telephone consultation. The telephone has become indispensable, and

Table 1.6   Barriers to Sustainability of Telemedicine Programs in the United States in 1996[24]

Barrier to sustainability	No. of programs	Percentage
Reimbursement	21	29.2
Telecom cost	11	15.3
General cost	9	12.5
Provider acceptance	6	8.3
Operating revenue	5	6.9
Organizational issues	3	4.2
Remote site commitment	3	4.2
Legal/regulatory	3	4.2

health care delivery systems as we know them could not exist without it. A brief review of the history of the telephone consultation gives insights into how other forms of telehealth might be effectively introduced into routine clinical practice. Interestingly, when physicians first used the telephone, they raised exactly the same objections to the technology as they now give about introducing telehealth.

USE OF THE TELEPHONE IN STANDARD MEDICAL PRACTICE FOR ADMINISTRATION AND CONSULTATION

We all now accept the telephone as a standard piece of medical equipment, just as we do the stethoscope,[25] so much so that in contemporary society health care could not be effectively delivered without it. For example, loss of emergency telephone service effectively cuts off the population from paramedic services. United States physicians make an average of 150 to 300 telephone calls a week directly associated with delivering patient care.[26] The area of patient care in which the telephone is used most often is delivering pediatric primary care services.[27–29] If telephone use for prescribing and getting test results are excluded, half of telephone consultations are undertaken to directly resolve a clinical problem.[30,31] One-sixth of ambulatory care visits have been replaced by a telephone call.[32] The telephone regularly substitutes for a direct visit in about one-third of office consultations, 1 in 50 home visits, and one-sixth of patient referrals made among hospital doctors. The pattern of health care delivery would be very different without patient and physician access to a telephone.

Although the telephone changes clinical practice, the nature of the clinical practice situation also affects the way in which the telephone is used in health care settings. Physicians' use of the telephone to practice clinically differs markedly between the United States and United Kingdom. Typically, only 7% of United Kingdom general practice consultations take place by telephone.[33] This difference relates to clinical practice because figures for rates of telephone use by United Kingdom general practices for general and administrative tasks are no different from those in other Western industrialized countries, whereas telephone consultation rates are much lower.[26] Reasons for this difference are unknown and are important for determining the growth potential for other forms of telehealth. It seems that referral mechanisms from primary care to the wider health care system are probably influential factors here, as well as different methods for payment/reimbursement. The availability of telephones and charges made for local telephone calls in the United Kingdom also may be contributory factors.

The Telephone Consultation: Who Consults and Why

For many patients the telephone consultation is often their entrée into the health care system. Data from primary care suggest 66% of patients call their doctors for reassurance, explanation of a worrying symptom, or advice. Sixteen percent of calls are for medication, and 7% are made because patients want to be seen immediately.[34] Typically, women are much more likely than men to call a doctor for a telephone consultation. There are, on average, 50 calls for every 100 male patients under 45 years of age per year.[35] This compares with an average of 170 calls per year for women over 65 years of age. The trigger initiating a telephone consultation is much more likely to relate to a definite symptom complex if the patient is either female or under 45 years old.[35,36] Common symptoms triggering a telephone consultation are shown in Table 1.7. In the United States, 9% of all drug prescribing for adults and up to 29% of prescribing for children take place over the telephone.[37]

The Accuracy and Content of Telephone Consultations

A physician can't directly examine a patient when using a conventional telephone to consult. When consulting with patients by telephone, physicians have to rely on verbal descriptions from patients, relatives, or other practitioners if they need to verify important physical findings such as tenderness at the site of pain and the appearance of any clinical abnormalities. Some physicians criticize the notion of videoconference consultations because they fear they will lose the vital dimension of a direct clinical examination. While accepting their concerns about this, we often find there are ambiguities of attitude and behavior when exploring their reasons. A clinician may summarily reject using interactive video for teleconsultation yet in exactly the same clinical situation will make decisions about whether to see a patient or to institute treatment remotely by using the telephone. Sixty percent of diagnoses in clinical medicine are made from the history alone. Intuitively, this suggests that, if an accurate history is taken, telephone and interactive videoconsultations should be equally safe and appropriate to use in deciding the initial management of appropriately selected patients.

The accuracy of clinical histories taken by clinicians over the telephone can vary widely.[38,39] When the accuracy of diagnosing otitis media (middle ear infections) by telephone is compared with the reliability of the same diagnosis made after a face-to-face consultation with the physician, 20% of the telephone cases are misdiagnosed.[40] This discrepancy in diagnosis may not be a consistent finding for all conditions because some clinical diagnoses are more dependent than others on direct physical examination of the patient

Table 1.7   Common Reasons for Patients Using the Telephone to Consult[26]

* Respiratory complaints
* Gastrointestinal problems
* Skin problems
* Fever
* Trauma

to verify or exclude specific findings. Making a definitive diagnosis of otitis media in a patient requires the direct visualization of a reddened eardrum. This dependency on a physical finding may be the reason for a discrepancy between the quality of diagnosis in telephone and face-to-face consultations. This is conjecture because it is unclear why there are differences.[40,41] Since the average telephone consultation can last 2–4 minutes,[42] lack of sufficient consultation time may be a contributory factor to misdiagnosis.

Physicians not only seem less competent in making a clinical diagnosis on the telephone; they also tend to make more precipitate diagnoses earlier in a consultation.[43,44] We believe this results from the fact that some clinicians inadvertently use a less rigorous approach to diagnosis over the telephone. Their telediagnostic approach assumes similar intuitions exist as in face-to-face consultations. Or they may be using stereotyped diagnostic methods to correct for the limitations of a telephone consultation. As physicians become more experienced in making a particular diagnosis, familiarity and time constraints make them reliant on diagnostic shortcuts based on intuition. These intuitions may work well in the face-to-face consultation because a physician unconsciously draws on a range of sensory cues as part of his/her diagnostic method. These cues are picked up from when the physician first sees the patient and they make eye contact. However, such supportive cues to diagnosis are absent on the telephone. Physicians who make diagnostic shortcuts in face-to-face consultations may adopt a similar approach to telephone consultation but do not make the necessary adjustments in their diagnostic reasoning for a lack of corroborative sensory information; hence, the poorer performance in consultation when using the telephone.

One way to correct the problem of misdiagnosis in telephone consultation is to work with clinical protocols/guidelines. Although it is still relatively uncommon for doctors to use protocols, paramedical professions increasingly use them to triage (decide how, when, and where to manage) patients.[45,46] Protocols are now widely used in most areas of health care. Their advantages to health care organizations are shown in Table 1.8. Clinical protocols/guidelines for telephone and interactive videoconsultations are

Table 1.8   Advantages of Using Clinical Protocols in Health Care

- Auditing clinical outcomes and reducing practice variation
- Reducing clinical risk
- Formalizing training
- Helping with billing and reimbursement
- Helping educate patients and inform them about what services are available

one way to ensure patients are consistently reviewed for direct physical examination and/or further investigation in situations where diagnostic errors are known to occur.

Training of Clinical Staff in the Telephone Consultation

Despite its importance in the delivery of health care, few physicians receive formal training on how to use the telephone effectively in clinical practice. Training in telephone consultation has not been a standard part of postgraduate medical training in the United Kingdom. In the United States, only 6% of internal medicine residencies offer basic training in how to manage patients over the telephone.[47] Where training on telephone consultation is provided, it amounts to only a single lecture in three fifths of programs and reading materials in half of programs. In the opinion of most residents, formal training in telephone management of their patients' problems is very important (62%), and they feel this training should form an integral part of every internal medicine curriculum (60%). Many practicing physicians recognize they have deficiencies when it comes to prescribing over the telephone.[48] Evidence for this as a major area of clinical risk in standard medical practice comes from the disturbing finding that four of every five health professionals could not clearly explain, in a way that patients could understand, how to take aspirin and acetaminophen for a fever when this information was given by them over the telephone.[38]

As yet we have no direct evidence training improves the standard of telephone consultation and will therefore result in better patient outcomes. Usually, when training programs offer help with telephone consultation, they concentrate on improving clinical history taking. They are making the assumption that this is the prime competency required for telephone consultation. In doing so they are simply transposing the construct of traditional clinical history taking onto telehealth as if it must be the "ideal" model to use for teleconsultation. Although it is an intuitive assumption, it ignores the possibility there may be distinct aspects to telephone consultation in particular and telehealth in general requiring the development of new models of consultation. The traditional clinical method used by most physicians is based on the doctor acting as an agent to elicit information. The model does not allow patients to assume the role of consumers who can seek information for themselves and make their own health care decisions.

A Customer-Based Approach to Telephone Consultation?

A customer-oriented approach asks patients what they want from their health care system and compares this with what they then actually complain to their physician about. Marked differences exist between this and conventional practice.[49] Reassurance, explanation, and advice are what patients value most from an after-hours telephone consultation with a physician.[50] It seems as though patients use the telephone to organize their thoughts and develop strategies to help deal with specific physical and/or emotional symptoms. They're uncertain about the significance of physical and emotional symptoms. Patients and physicians can therefore approach consultations from different standpoints. The patient is often unsure about what is happening and wants to establish whether a problem is significant, regardless of whether the physician knows exactly what is wrong. A problem must be real for a patient if it is important enough for him/her to overcome the usual hurdles to getting consultation time with a physician. Physicians are conditioned to analyze symptoms and establish diagnoses. Physicians are often looking for certainty whereas the patient wants to explore the uncertainty. In such exploratory situations there are three prime features underlying a successful teleconsultation:

1. *Listen closely to what the patient is actually complaining of.* This means the physician must not only listen to the words themselves but also to the way a patient speaks them. Inflection of the voice, together with timbre and tone, are cues to helping the physician sense whether the minor physical ailment complained of is the real or the ostensible reason for the consultation. Is this what the patient is using to establish a preliminary rapport with the physician before she/he confides a more serious concern such as violence, abuse, or fear of cancer?

2. *Provide the direct care that is appropriate to what the patient is complaining of.* If the patient complains of central chest pain with pain radiating down the left arm, a wise physician will want to examine the patient further and investigate him/her to exclude a heart attack. The teleconsultation may therefore have a variety of possible purposes. It may be a closed consultation with a problem recognized, the problem dealt with, and then the patient discharged with no follow-up. Conversely, the teleconsultation may be no

more than an initial method of triage, with the eventual outcome required being a face-to-face consultation or a referral elsewhere for additional specialist advice.

3.   *Health education advice.* If the patient's complaint is of a hoarse voice present for a few hours after attending a football match, the appropriate advice may be to watch and wait because it may be a temporary effect from too much shouting. The wise physician will cover "what if" scenarios; for example, what if the hoarseness does not go within a specified time because the patient may have an underlying throat cancer and the shouting is just a red herring?

When using the telephone the physician should always err on the side of seeing a patient or referring him/her somewhere else for further advice if there is diagnostic doubt.[45] The purpose of a telephone consultation is therefore not necessarily to establish absolute certainty about a situation. Often it is to gauge the extent of a patient's uncertainty and then help make a decision about what is best to do.

GENERAL LESSONS FOR TELEHEALTH FROM THE RECENT HISTORY OF TELEMEDICINE AND FROM A CENTURY OF TELEPHONE CONSULTATION

Recent experience with telemedicine and telephone consultation suggests the major challenge confronting the adoption of telehealth by health care organizations may not be associated with only the technology or its cost. Instead, it may be how readily people can adapt to using the new technology in practice. Telehealth invariably means changes in clinical practice. There are two reasons for this. First, change in practice is often required to make the cost savings needed to justify an initial investment in telehealth. Second, the nature of teleconsultations differs from face-to-face consultations, and clinicians must adapt the way they practice to accommodate this difference. Accepting telehealth challenges clinicians to change their accepted ways of practicing their profession, so they and the professional organizations representing them are understandably concerned about telehealth and its possible effects on the standard of care.

Anecdotal experience suggests a major, often unstated fear among clinicians is of a future in which clinical practice is spent in front of a television screen or visual display unit (VDU). We cannot absolutely assure them this fear is unjustified. However, the introduction of the telephone was associated with similar fears on the part of many physicians. Our prediction is that telehealth will never remove the need for face-to-face clinical consultation between health care practitioners and patients. Telehealth programs regularly mention instances of patients who are prepared to travel for many hours for a face-to-face clinical consultation despite the availability of telehealth because they intrinsically value the face-to-face consultation. Our mainstay of practical reassurance to clinicians who voice concerns about telehealth is that they trust in the basic strength of the face-to-face consultation. This may change but is most unlikely to go away with telehealth. Some reluctance among clinicians toward telehealth is natural. Clinicians held similar misgivings in the past toward the stethoscope and the telephone. Inevitably each of these technologies was successfully introduced. In retrospect no one would seriously advocate that the use of either of these should have been abolished. In the future we believe resistance to telehealth will be looked back on with the same wonderment as we feel about concerns over the use of the stethoscope. Because of these fears it is important telehealth programs have clear and a decisive lead from clinicians in their implementation plans.

We believe it is vital for clinician leaders to engage in defining the future of telehealth. Strategic planning of telehealth programs always requires clinical perspectives as well as system and cost considerations. If a realistic clinical input is not included in telehealth strategies, cost factors alone will decide. A century of telephone consultation offers lessons for devising what should be included in the clinical components of new telehealth applications, as shown in Table 1.9.

The traditional face-to-face doctor-patient interaction is often taken by some as a gold standard compared to which a telehealth consultation is inferior. Areas of unreliability in both conventional face-to-face consultation and telephone consultations raise questions about the best way to structure a telehealth consultation. Telehealth programs often seem to view telehealth as merely an assembly of various technological tools, such as a camera and remote stethoscope to which clinician and patient are attached and which reproduces conventional methods of clinical practice. We agree in part with this approach; however, this method risks losing elements of the humanity of care and diagnostic accuracy, particularly if the necessary research and training are not carried out to support the change in practice. An overwhelming lesson learned when telephone consultations were introduced was how training of clinicians was neglected. Even today telephone consultation is a major unrecognized area of clinical risk in most medical practice. It is important telehealth does not blindly follow suit. We strongly advocate training programs in telehealth be based on protocols/guidelines into which *evidence of clinical effectiveness* is incorporated where available.

Table 1.9   Lessons from Telephone Consultation for Telehealth

- Normal methods of clinical consultation do not automatically transpose into teleconsultations.
- The aims and objectives of the teleconsulation must be clearly established.
- There is a definite place for the use of clinical protocols in teleconsultation.
- Clinicians, no matter how experienced in conventional practice, need training and education in methods of teleconsultation.
- Enough time must be prioritized to teleconsultation; otherwise mistakes can be made.
- Clinicians must learn to reorient their thinking toward exploring uncertainty, not establishing a certain diagnosis, if they are going to use teleconsultation safely in routine clinical practice.

Properly formulated and introduced, clinical guidelines and protocols retain the best of the humanity and diagnostic accuracy of conventional practice and remove unacceptable variations in clinical practice. The use of practice guidelines and protocols is a contentious area in health care, particularly for physicians who feel that these threaten their freedom of clinical practice. Although this is a legitimate concern, we believe telehealth must use these tools to add structure, discipline, and systematization to the teleconsultation. An airline pilot who is responsible for the lives of several hundred people on an airplane would be considered negligent if she/he flew the airplane without having protocols to check the integrity and function of the controls and instruments. Airplane crash investigations repeatedly show how pilot error is the cause of airplane crashes in 70% of cases. We strongly advocate the development of clinical guidelines and protocols before using teleconsultation in routine clinical practice. Reasons why guidelines/protocols are necessary in telehealth are given in Table 1.10.

It is not enough to just develop these clinical protocols/guidelines for telehealth. Clinicians must have adequate training and education to help them use telehealth systems effectively and appropriately. They need to learn the basics of why, when, and how they should teleconsult. Expecting clinicians to be skilled in teleconsultation simply because they have practiced conventional medicine is a dangerous assumption. Acquiring new clinical skills in medicine once used to consist of following a pattern of "see one, do one, teach one." This method is no longer acceptable because it means mistakes in learning are made on patients. The known deficiencies in the telephone consultation are warnings not to take this retrogressive approach to telehealth. The time to establish a culture of training and professionalism in telehealth consultations is right at the outset, when establishing the program. If this is not done, loose practice and bad habits can become ingrained, as they have with telephone consultation. The best way to establish the

Table 1.10   Reasons Why Guidelines/Protocols Are Necessary in Telehealth

- To monitor the quality of health care services provided using telehealth
- To establish consistent training programs for practitioners in using telehealth
- For clinical contracting for telehealth
- For clinical risk and claims management in telehealth
- To give clear and unambiguous information to patients about telehealth services for reassurance and to promote their use of these services
- For effective management of telehealth services

framework for training and education in telehealth is to use guidelines and protocols developed by the clinicians who are actually teleconsulting. Telehealth programs can support clinicians in developing guidelines by establishing a culture to support setting standards, devising protocols/guidelines, and instituting training and education. These processes require more than goodwill. They require management expertise and resourcing if they are to happen.

2

Telehealth: A Patient Perspective

How well telehealth providers respond to the demands and expectations their patients place on remote care delivery systems is critical to the future of remotely delivered health care. One of telehealth's main strengths is its capacity to help make health care systems consumer-friendly. We contend that health care systems are not, nor ever have been, particularly consumer-friendly. They are now set on a new and changed course because of

- Pressure from legislation and regulation by government
- Patients' demands
- The dictates of market-based health care systems

The US and UK governments seem to have relinquished central planning of service delivery as a way to shape health care systems. Consumer pressure from employers and the general public, who pay for health care services, as well as from the patients who receive these services, is playing an ever increasing role in shaping the configuration of our health care systems. Government has adopted the position of trying to influence the outputs or outcomes of health care systems as a way to shape their future rather than trying to micromanage the process of care delivery itself. We look at measuring the clinical outputs of health care processes in a later chapter on evidence-based health care. In this chapter we will consider outputs of the health care system in terms of the rights, roles, and expectations of patients.

Attempts to formalize the rights of patients as consumers of health care services, include the Patients' Bill of Rights in the United States and the Patients' Charter initiative introduced previously in the United Kingdom. Health care consumerism in different forms of expression may mold the future of health care in the United Kingdom, United States, New Zealand, Australia, and Canada. All these countries appear set on approximately convergent courses toward a mixed public/private provision of health care. In one sense the only differences among them lie in the exact entitlements to and exclusions from health care in the public and private sectors in each. In all these countries telehealth will play a major role in how health care delivery is restructured by helping define patient (consumer) rights, roles, and expectations in ways this chapter describes.

THE IMPORTANCE OF A PATIENT FOCUS FOR TELEHEALTH

The growth strategy of many telehealth service providers has been to market and sell their products directly to large health care provider organizations. Their view in doing so assumes health care providers (usually large hospitals) are the main customers for telehealth products, not patients. Many of the senior executives in large hospitals seem to view patients as predominantly a source of income for their institution, not as educated consumers with preferences to express and choices to make. Consequently, the patient perspective is rarely considered when deciding if, when, and how to introduce telehealth into a health care environment. Instead, large health care provider organizations are frequently preoccupied with three concerns:

◆ Their large fixed-capital assets (usually hospitals). These are becoming increasingly inappropriate for their core business activities. This concern forces a health care provider to focus on servicing their major capital asset instead of the needs of the patients passing through it as entitled consumers.

◆ A relatively inflexible labor force that usually reacts negatively to inevitable changes (e.g., consumerism in health care or changes in clinical practice associated with introducing telehealth systems cost-effectively).

◆ Senior management teams that are reactive, not proactive, to inevitable change, such as consumer pressure in health care. This often links to the understandable need to focus on quarterly financial performance figures. Such indices do not equate to patients' experiences as consumers in the current health care environment—a situation that attempts to legislate on patients' rights are trying to address.

So although the boardroom of a large hospital may physically resemble its counterparts in industry and commerce outside, and although many of its financial and internal management processes are comparable, there is usually one striking difference. In today's competitive markets, senior executives in commerce and industry have to focus obsessively on what their customers want. Attention to their customers' needs permeates all their strategic thinking and most management actions. This behavior contrasts starkly with the low premium some health care organizations currently place on the preferences of patients. It is not unknown for board meetings in major health care organizations to run their course and mention the word *patient* only as a statistical index of projected variances in expected revenues. In doing this they ignore

- Whether patients could have participated in any of the changes under consideration.
- How patients may be affected by the decisions being made.
- The fact that concerns about patients as consumers could determine all or part of the meeting's agenda.

When senior management teams in health care organizations ignore patient preferences, the rest of the organization inevitably follows this lead. In many ways the attitude toward patients as consumers in some health care organizations is reminiscent of how industrial and commercial companies outside health care treated consumers until a decade ago. Today's successful industrial and commercial companies not only talk about what their consumers want; they actively take steps to find out what they want. No competently managed company thinks of launching a new product line without first market testing and getting a detailed analysis of consumer preferences. Painful experiences in the late 1980s and early 1990s taught companies the lesson of how perilous it is to ignore their consumers. Against the current backdrop of industry, how health care organizations behave toward patients seems a curious anomaly in today's consumer-oriented societies.

Consumerism offers people the option of looking elsewhere when they are unhappy with any goods or services on offer. A major problem for patients as consumers of health care has been the lack of information about services—information they need to make informed choices. A precondition for markets to work is free access to information for consumers. This deficiency is diminishing as an ever-growing number of people now access information about health care services from Internet sites.[51,52] The burgeoning number of these on-line information resources is making patients aware of the following long-standing inconsistencies in relation to their health care services:

- ◆ Patients' entitlements to health care vary according to where they live and what their health plan is.
- ◆ Physicians in the same specialty often treat people with the same condition differently for no apparent reason.
- ◆ These treatments are often unlinked to current scientific evidence.
- ◆ The results (outcomes) of a treatment may vary widely according to where the treatment was given.
- ◆ The amount patients pay for health care services may depend on where they are treated.
- ◆ There is not necessarily a correlation between the amount paid for treatment and the results subsequently obtained in terms of improved health.

A self-educated minority of patients who now use the Internet regularly for information about health care is discovering something health care professionals have always known. There are major inequities in who gets access to health care services and also wide variations in the quality of the care provided for those who do have access to services.[53,54] "Internet-wise" patients are now beginning to exercise their rights as informed consumers and are expecting to get the best-quality health care at a fair price. Will they continue to passively accept complacent and discriminatory attitudes toward them from health care systems they ultimately pay for? This must be a largely rhetorical question because they would not tolerate these discriminatory attitudes in any other aspect of their lives. The implications of educated and informed groups of patients for telehealth are therefore as follows:

- ◆ Telehealth on the Internet is already a major change agent in a rapidly growing movement toward a consumer focus in health care.
- ◆ Organizations interested in providing telehealth must adopt a patient focus if they are going to capitalize on the opportunities telehealth offers.
- ◆ There may be major financial risks associated with introducing a telehealth program and ignoring the growing dynamic of informed patients acting as consumers.

HOW THE CHANGING ROLE OF THE PATIENT INFLUENCES TELEHEALTH

Consumer pressure and new technology have transformed the societies in which we live. Many large factories have closed down, giving way to smaller and more flexible workplaces. Similarly, many city center department stores have transformed themselves in response to consumer pressure for stores in more convenient malls. There was a clear rationale in the industrial age to concentrate capital investment, achieve economies of scale, and focus processes in large institutions. The large factory, the department store, and the hospital were prime examples of these large Victorian-inspired institutions. Are these appropriate for the information age? Alone among these large institutions the hospital seems to survive unscathed.

Times are changing. Social infrastructures must adapt and gear themselves up to support postindustrial societies. The disadvantages of hospitals for patients are that they

- May necessitate traveling long distances to get treatment.
- Separate patients from relatives and friends.
- Institutionalize patients into set regimens governing waking, dressing, eating, visiting, and sleeping.
- Not only concentrate resources and patients but also microorganisms (there are substantial risks to patients of acquiring infections in a hospital).
- Seem an increasingly expensive way to deliver health care in an environment of scarce resources.

Telehealth can significantly contribute toward making the Victorian-inspired institution of the hospital into a more consumer-friendly place for patients. Hospitals are important for the delivery of health care and are likely to remain so in the future. As with factories and shops, hospitals now face pressure to adapt. Telehealth offers ways of providing locally accessible, consumer-friendly services. A growing dilemma for telehealth providers is whether to keep concentrating their marketing effort toward large hospital providers as their key clients. These sales strategies are often based on selling relatively low volumes of high-cost equipment. Part of the societal drive for change away from department stores and factories reflect how high-volume, low-cost sales strategies cater to consumer demand. Telehealth providers could therefore base their sales and marketing strategies on increasing their sales in the primary care sector and in the primary/secondary care interface instead of their traditional reliance on the large hospital. Telehealth enables specialist consultation and high-tech health care applications such as dermatology and cardiology to become accessible to patients in primary care. Patients are then able to receive these services near home instead of having to travel to a hospital. In promoting these changes, telehealth inevitably affects the culture and work practices of health care organizations.

When specialist health services are delivered through primary care, health care professionals often have to alter how, when, and where they work. Encouraging consumer pressure forces hospitals to adapt and can therefore mean that health care professionals face disruptions to their work practice similar to those that factory and department store workers experienced when the forces of change affected them. The resulting flexibility of labor markets in commerce and industry increased productivity and helped reduce the cost of consumer goods. Telehealth offers the real promise of making the same kinds of cost savings in health care, as we will attempt to show later. When looking at telehealth, health purchasers want to find these same benefits as one way to combat the continued rise in health care costs. For telehealth to deliver these cost savings and make health care services more consumer-focused requires responsive contracting to redirect resources. In doing so, telehealth runs even greater risk of antagonizing health care professional groups.

Telehealth providers must make strategic decisions about how they want to relate to patients as consumers of health care, and clearly there are risks associated with choosing to relate more closely to patients. This strategy can potentially alienate them from their existing client base in health care. Looking at comparative rates of consultation in health care provides a strong argument in favor of adoption by telehealth providers of a greater focus on patients. Most telehealth programs have disappointingly low rates of patient teleconsultation, and this has important consequences for revenue projections in their business. Low rates of teleconsultation threaten their prospects for long-term survival, as we will describe later. Interestingly, an area of telehealth with a phenomenal growth in the number of patients accessing new services has been consumer health information sites on the Internet. Many purists in the field of telemedicine would exclude Internet health information sites from their definition of telemedicine, but they clearly lie within our definition of telehealth.

Such a demand for health information on the Internet is not surprising. Energetic, vocal, and inquiring groups of people are getting that do not fit with past stereotypes of patients on-line health information. We hear patients in focus groups express their feelings about how health care organizations treat them, with statements such as

- "As patients we are expected to have things done to us."
- "We feel that we have to accept what we are told without being able to question."
- "It is not that we have a problem with the care we receive. We just want to know what is happening to us and why."

+ "With work, homes, and families it is just so inconvenient to get to the hospital, with the travel, parking, waiting, and uncertainty about what is going to happen."

In statements like these, patients are showing that, as health care consumers, they want their experiences to mirror their expectations as consumers in other areas of their life. These feelings do not fit with traditional ideas about the role of the patient. In recognition of this, other terms, such as "users of health care" and "health care consumers," have been used to capture this sense of giving people more involvement in deciding what health care they want to receive and how they want it delivered. These descriptions have not caught on because patients, the general public, and health care professionals are unhappy with them. The response from focus groups of patients is that they have no problem with the word *patient;* what they object to is the label of passivity it currently implies. They want this image to change.

In not recognizing the legitimacy and importance of Internet-based health care information a telemedicine program fails to acknowledge the interests of patients as consumers. Such programs are continuing the emphasis on the "delivery of care *to*" not the "provision of services *for* patients." Supportive evidence to suggest lack of a patient focus in the strategic thinking of telemedicine programs comes from the dearth of data on patient views in the telemedicine literature. This literature now amounts to several thousand professional journal articles and books on telehealth/telemedicine published since 1966.[55,56] If telehealth programs focus predominantly on the technology, clinical process, and finance rather than on patients, it is no surprise to find telehealth programs with several million dollars invested in equipment that are to attract only a few hundred patient consultations per year.

Low rates of teleconsultation are causing many telehealth organizations to revisit their original development strategy and wonder if they miscalculated. They invested heavily in establishing elaborate infrastructures to support what health care organizations and physicians wanted to deliver to patients but did not do market research to find out what patients want and need. Epidemiological data on the incidence and prevalence of disease can help to define the "needs" of patients (e.g., in terms of dermatological, cardiological, and ophthalmological disease, etc.). What these epidemiological approaches frequently forget to gather data on is what patients repeatedly ask for—information. Health care systems around the world are using market mechanisms to allocate health care resources. A basic precondition necessary to allow markets to work effectively is ensuring that consumers have access to information about the goods and services available.

The changes we are seeing in the character of patients is that they are acting as informed consumers who demand access to information about the health care they receive. This is precisely what a market system for health care should demand. Meeting this escalating demand for patient information is a major growth area for telehealth worldwide. Growth rates in this sector of telehealth, one predominantly based on the Internet and other broadcast media, far outstrip those in telehealth delivery programs, into which the vast majority of time, energy, and money have been placed but so far with a disappointing return on investment. Who provides health care information to patients, or health care consumers, is of major strategic importance to the future development of telehealth and also to the future evolution of health care systems worldwide.

TELEHEALTH AND PROVIDING HEALTH INFORMATION TO CONSUMERS

The major initial thrust for providing organized health care information for patients/consumers via telehealth came from government agencies. The US government has a Healthfinder Web site (www.healthfinder.gov),[57] a place where any interested person can get general health care information. A range of other US government agencies now provides information that consumers can access on-line, including

- The Food and Drug Administration (FDA)[58]
- Health Care Financing Administration (HCFA), the Medicare and Medicaid agency[59]
- U.S. Department of Health and Human Services[60]

In addition to these governmental examples, a diverse range of organizations interested in health care issues supports growing numbers of Internet Web sites. The *1997 Healthcare Guide to the Internet*[61] enumerates over 500 Internet sites where health care information is available. New health information sites are coming on-line daily. As of late 1999 there were over 24,000 health-related Internet Web sites.

If they align themselves exclusively with health care providers, telehealth programs can find themselves locked into "closed" information systems. These closed systems are the proprietary information systems of the health care provider, and they usually concentrate on providing clinical information and clinical services for practitioners to deliver to patients. A down side for a telehealth provider of these closed systems is that it is difficult for them to operate as primary providers of health information to patients. Patients are eager for information and so seek out places outside telehealth programs to find it. Significant numbers of patients turn to the Internet as their primary information source when making health care decisions. This change is a significant fragmentation of the market for telehealth. Instead of telehealth systems offering health information and delivering care, these functions may have already become irretrievably split.

In the United States, where the health care system is more strongly market-driven than elsewhere, health plans and health maintenance organizations (HMOs) clearly recognize the growing demand of patients for information and the strategic importance this has for their businesses. Health plans that have been reluctant to invest in telehealth systems to deliver health care are rushing to establish and maintain Internet Web sites. Initially, these sites have been information resources for their subscribers, helping them to access details of their health coverage and general health information.[62,63] Increasingly, HMOs are developing Web sites to give general health promotion advice and coverage information to their members.[64] Why are health plans and HMOs so eager to get into providing consumer health information to patients using the Internet?

Health plans and HMOs are investing in the Internet provision of health care information because it offers them a direct link to their consumers. In contrast to health care providers, health care purchasers have been desperate to find ways to engage in dialogues with their subscribers and help make them informed health care consumers. Until the general population was able to access the Internet, there was no easy way for health plans, insurers, and government agencies purchasing health care to reach out directly to canvass patients' views. Postal or face-to-face surveys of patients and the general population were the only reliable ways to get information about patients' expectations and satisfaction in the recent past. Surveys such as these are expensive, and their value is often time-limited to the date when the original survey data were collected. This has meant that the main routine source of information on what patients feel about the health care they receive has often been what individual physicians and health care provider organizations offered. Information sources have consisted largely of the "I know what my patients want" type of data and are therefore subject to major sources of bias. The value of Internet connectivity to their consumers for a health plan or HMO is precisely that it can verify uncorroborated assertions from health care providers who "know what [their] patients want."

The difficulty of disentangling what patients may actually want from what hospitals and physicians say they want is a crucial issue in health care consumerism. Decisions dependent on knowing what is good for patients can become inextricably linked to what is thought to be good for practitioners and hospitals. Health care purchasers want to know firsthand what their patients want and then use this information to make decisions, for example about introducing innovations like telehealth. In a cost-conscious health care environment they will introduce a new intervention such as telehealth only if it

+ Is of proven clinical effectiveness.
+ Reduces the costs of care or improves clinical quality at the same price.
+ Is acceptable to patients.

Health care purchasers find it difficult to change the way services are delivered because of the professional and organizational barriers they must overcome. If the barriers to telehealth's widespread introduction are overcome, they see telehealth as a potential tool to help break the cycle of ever-increasing health care costs. Some states in the United States and provinces in Canada have already established state/province-wide telehealth systems to deliver health care. These investments were often made with an explicit expectation that health care costs could be reduced. As yet it is unclear how these programs will capture a patient perspective and use this to influence health care purchasing decisions. These telehealth initiatives commonly take place using real-time videoconsultation and store-and-forward teleconsultations on closed information systems, where access is limited to practitioners and does not include a direct feedback loop from patients.

Teletriage using the telephone is one proven area of telehealth where engaging in a dialogue with a patient as a consumer reduces health care utilization and therefore costs.[46] Teletriage enables patients with acute health problems to contact a nurse by telephone, discuss their condition, and get help and information. The nurse directs the patient to the most appropriate place for care, using clinical protocols. The UK government introduced plans to make teletriage available throughout the National Health Service (NHS) as part of its 1997 White Paper proposals for health care reorganization. It is seen as an easily implemented measure to improve quality and reduce the costs of health care delivery. Health plans and governments are eager to explore various ways of creating links to patients as health care consumers using real-time videoconferencing, store-and-forward, and E-mail.

The use of the telephone for teletriage has raised some other interesting issues for telehealth. Equity of access for their populations to health care services is a concern most governments want to address. Although the percentage of households with computers is rising in the United States and the United Kingdom as prices of systems drop, for the immediate future there will be "haves" and "have nots" as defined in terms of which individuals and families have ready access to cyberspace. Aside from any political and ethical considerations, this development has caused health plans, HMOs, and health care purchasers such as HCFA to face more mundane, practical considerations. Currently using the Internet to provide information about services, eligibility, and health benefits to patients means double-running existing paper and telephone information services alongside the new Internet service. This duplication often means telehealth increases costs in the short term until enough of the population can access the new service and older information delivery systems can be dropped. Although there are important issues to be resolved, we believe the Internet is now an intertwined part of the future configuration of health care services, as shown in Figure 2.1. This figure illustrates how Internet Web sites can feed into databases providing information to health care purchasers about patients and supplement traditional sources of information from health care providers.

From this discussion it should not be inferred government and health care purchasers have the exclusive interest in using the Internet to communicate with health care consumers. Health care providers, drug companies, and health care equipment and appliance manufacturers are equally interested in the possibilities the Internet has to offer. Health care providers are establishing Web sites to link directly with patients.[65,66] The patient-associated reasons that hospitals are linking to the Internet are

- Marketing of their services.
- Giving information about directions and clinic times.
- Obtaining patient feedback for quality assurance.

Suddenly, instead of a dearth of information for patients, *everybody*—government, purchasers of health care, hospitals, physicians' groups, individual physicians, drug companies, and medical equipment suppliers—are all getting into the business of giving information to patients. New sources of health information are already bringing with them problems as well as benefits. Patients may see their physicians with seven or more pages of information from the Internet. Patients with this information expect their physicians to assimilate the information, synthesize it, and then incorporate it into a recommendation about treatment within the constraints of a 15-minute consultation. Data overload can thereby transform the once sought after Holy Grail of health information into sludge blocking the health care delivery process. For health information to work effectively, the patient/practitioner consultation must adapt. Either more consultation time is required or the information must be provided in a readily exchangeable currency for patient

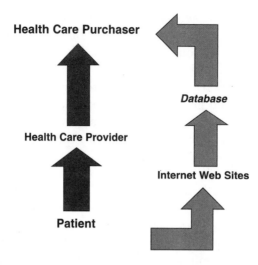

Figure 2.1   The flow of information from patient to purchasers of health care using the Internet.

and practitioner to use in negotiating the optimum health care treatment options. Altering the doctor-patient relationship to make telehealth work is a complex organizational change process that is frequently overlooked in telehealth programs. We consider this point in chapter 3.

Once the process is started, providing reliable, robust, and accurate health care information on the Internet can become an expensive ongoing commitment for an organization. Keeping the information content fresh and relevant for consumers is a costly and time-consuming aspect of maintaining a Web site. From the health care consumers' perspective, no fool-proof mechanisms exist to help them make judgments about the quality, accuracy, and safety of the health-related information they see posted on the Internet. We predict a rapid growth of health information sites on the Internet, posting information in the form of consumer reports to help patients assimilate and understand the issues confronting them in making health care decisions. How these patient information resources will be funded long-term and will manage to navigate the treacherous medicolegal minefield remains to be worked out.

In the meantime, health information on the Internet will continue to create problems. Sources for the data provided are often not given on Web sites. All too often, therefore, "seeing has to be believing" for health-related information on the Internet. With the exponential growth of health care information on the Internet, what was a relative famine of information is rapidly becoming a medieval-style banquet of health-associated data. Key issues being thrown from this table are

+ What information patients want about health care and who should provide this.
+ What information health care purchasers want from patients and what information they need to give in return.
+ What information health care providers want from patients and what they want to communicate back to patients.
+ How the quality of health-related information can be judged in order to use it effectively.

WHAT INFORMATION DO PATIENTS WANT ABOUT HEALTH CARE?

Patients say they are unhappy at the small amount of information they receive from doctors and hospitals about their health care problems and the way they receive it. How much information to give patients and when and how to give it to them are complex dynamics. Individual clinicians often insist they are the best judges of what information their patients want and when to provide it. The following anecdotal clinical story shows how difficult it can be to take this assertion at face value (A. Darkins, personal communication, 1987):

A patient was referred from his own physician. The physician's referral letter read:

Mr. _____ is a 68-year-old retired car worker with inoperable lung cancer. He has severe midthoracic back pain. I am concerned about the possibility of a secondary deposit in his spine. Could you please advise what are the risks of spinal cord compression and of the possible treatment options, including simple palliation for the pain? Mr. _____ is unaware of his diagnosis or of the prognosis. I would be grateful if you would not tell him either of these because I don't believe he is capable of handling this information.

Mr. _____ came into the consulting room, and the first thing he said after sitting down was "Doctor, I know have cancer of the lung and I am going to die soon. My own doctor has a problem with talking with me about this. I have bad pain in my back, and I want to know what this means and what you can do to make this easier so that I can sleep at night."

This anecdote illustrates one of the real dilemmas in giving information to patients in clinical medicine. Who should make clinical decisions affecting an individual's life and well-being? Should the physician make the decision? Should the patient? Should they decide jointly? These are pertinent questions relating to the implementation of a new telehealth service. Real-time teleconsultation could mean the two clinicians in the clinical anecdote above might be videoconsulting with the patient present throughout. Unless clear understandings about who makes decisions are agreed on, unsightly and unprofessional disagreements could erupt, with the patient caught in the middle. Developments such as health care consumerism and telehealth make the person associated with the disease at least as important as the disease itself.

Until recently, the major emphasis of medical education was on understanding the natural history of diseases, not how these diseases affected patients' lives. A major step forward in understanding the part patient preferences can play in clinical decision making came from the work done by Jack Wennberg, an epidemiologist from New Hampshire, and associates such as Michael Barry and Al Mulley, both physicians from Massachusetts. They and others were instrumental in developing the Shared Decision-making Program (SDP) for patients and doctors[67] to use as a decision-support tool in routine consultations.

The SDP originated in the United States in the late 1980s and involved giving patients information about the risks and benefits of treatments for common conditions, including the following:

- Benign prostate disease
- Mild hypertension
- Breast cancer
- Low back pain
- Prostate cancer
- Hormone replacement therapy
- Benign uterine conditions
- Ischemic heart disease

Using a multimedia platform, the SDP profoundly changed thinking about how to give clinical information to patients. It emphasized patients' rights to ownership of decisions affecting their health and longevity. The SDP program helped in clarifying the subjects patients want information about:

- What is their condition and how has it arisen?
- How does their condition affect their health?
- What does their condition mean in terms of their chances of living or dying?

- What is the natural history of their condition if untreated?
- What is the likelihood of a cure for their condition if treated?
- What treatment options are available?
- What are the benefits of treatment?
- What are the risks associated with treatment?
- What is the likelihood of their receiving benefit from treatment?
- What is the likelihood of their suffering a complication of the treatment?
- What things suggest that their condition is worsening?
- What things suggest that their condition is improving?

Involving patients directly in the decisions about their care often requires different information from what previous experience and intuition might predict. The SDP program illustrated this well in relation to giving men information about benign prostate disease (J. Wennberg, M. Barry, & A. Mullen, personal communication, 1992). When men come for advice about surgery for benign prostate disease, doctors often fail to routinely give them information about prostate cancer. The physician may not want to bother the man with the unpleasantness of mentioning the possibility of cancer, or the physician may see it as irrelevant when the disease is probably benign. Giving information about prostate cancer to patients who are considering surgery for benign prostate disease is important for the following two reasons:

1. A small percentage of patients who seem to have benign prostate disease before operation turn out to have prostate cancer when a pathological analysis of the prostate gland material is done after operation. It can cause more distress to be told after a prostate operation that cancer has been found instead of being prewarned of the possibility beforehand.

2. Some men imagine that surgery on their prostate gland for benign prostate disease removes all chance of their getting prostate cancer later. Therefore, these men are tempted to have prostate surgery (a prostatectomy) whether they believe their current symptoms warrant it or not. They think that prostatectomy is analogous to the removal of the uterus in a woman with benign uterine disease, which eliminates the risk of uterine cancer, but this is not the case with prostatectomy for benign prostate disease. The most common operation (transurethral resection of the prostate [TURP]) undertaken for benign prostatic hypertrophy leaves a rim of prostate tissue against the capsule (outside) of the prostate gland, a place where prostate cancer commonly arises. The risk of prostate cancer remains after a TURP and should not therefore be a factor in a man's decision about whether or not to have prostate surgery for benign prostate disease.

The SDP gave information about the outcomes of health care to patients using interactive video technology and was another example of using telehealth in routine clinical practice. The concept underlying the SDP was to provide decision support to patients, enabling them and their doctors to use information about the outcomes of treatment jointly to make health care decisions. After the original pioneering work of the SDP there has been an explosion of interest in exploring ways to give clinical information to patients and help them with decision making. The reasons underlying this interest include the following

- Improving the quality of health care
- Reducing health care utilization rates
- Business opportunities in health care

Various media are being used to provide this information, including the Internet, interactive video, videocassette, and computer programs. The challenge for companies and projects active in this area of multimedia is how to get uptake of clinical decision-support tools into the doctor–patient interaction and so make them more widely available to patients. The SDP and other projects helped in showing the nature of the health information patients want to obtain. The ongoing challenge for telehealth is how to combine health information delivery platforms with the process of delivering health care and so provide information acceptable to both physicians and patients.

VERIFYING THE INFORMATION GIVEN PATIENTS IN TELEHEALTH PROGRAMS

In an information age, where telehealth is now regularly used to give information to patients, there are two important components to assemble and link into processes for delivering care. One component is the technology necessary to deliver information and the second is the information itself. Information is not a value-free commodity, and finding clinical information that patients and physicians both understand and agree on is an essential part of making it a tool for the joint negotiation of clinical decisions. Providers of health care information to patients typically include the following:

- Health care providers
- Health care purchasers
- Patient organizations
- Drug companies
- Medical equipment suppliers

- Government agencies
- Private foundations
- Private individuals
- Internet providers
- Publishers of newspapers, magazines, and books
- Television and cable networks

As mentioned earlier, the sheer volume of information available can lead to information overload. How do physicians and patients judge the quality of information they use to make clinical decisions? Not all providers of health information have pure motives in making this information available. Where does information providing end and marketing of a health care product, service, or drug begin? Where are patients to go for unbiased information about health care?

Central governments are shrinking away from directly managing health care services. They leave these decisions to the market. Increasingly, they see their role as one of setting policy, monitoring standards, and overseeing how outcome information is provided in health care systems. Worldwide there is a move toward collecting evidence on the effectiveness of treatments used in health care. The Canadian government sponsors major programs at McMaster University on evidence-based practice. The UK government established the Cochrane Center in the early 1990s, an organization with the original responsibility of collecting evidence of clinical effectiveness for use in the NHS. The Cochrane Center has since spawned a worldwide network focusing on clinical effectiveness. The US government has the Agency for Health Care Policy and Research (AHCPR) under whose auspices the Patient Outcome Research Team (PORT) work was accomplished.

All these initiatives have a common aim of producing information for doctors and patients about effective treatments. The gold standard of clinical effectiveness is the double-blind, randomized, controlled clinical trial. The US Preventive Services Task Force[68] produced a widely used tool to assess the quality of scientific evidence of literature on the effectiveness of treatments. Unfortunately, scientific evidence about clinical effectiveness is not usually in an easily palatable form for either clinicians or patients to digest. The UK government established a dissemination center for information on clinical effectiveness, based in York, to find solutions to this problem.

Despite the good intentions of these and other initiatives, the weight of support in the clinical consultation lies firmly behind the practitioner. Clinicians have a vast armamentarium of clinical support tools to make decisions for patients, such as x-ray and biochemical tests. So far, evidence-based medicine initiatives seem to have directed their emphasis more toward the clinician than the patient. If the clinical information patients receive is to be useful and nego-tiable, not resulting in giving seven pages of Internet material to their physi-cian to read in a consultation, more emphasis must be placed on informing the patient. Telehealth systems should look toward giving patients "evidence-based *choice*,"[69] not just "evidence-based medicine." A major challenge for telehealth is therefore to set up the collaborations and alliances necessary to develop the intellectual products that patients and practitioners require if they are going to make decisions together in the rapidly changing world of health care.

A related challenge is how patients are going to access information from telehealth providers. Internet service providers are increasingly moving toward developing portals through which people will access a range of related products and services. Although it is not clear how these portals will operate nor how improved search engines on the Internet will affect such develop-ments, we believe it would hamper the development of telehealth if func-tionally closed systems developed on the Internet. The stock market value of a portal is often based on expected revenues from advertising sold to catch the patient in cyberspace. Although the entrepreneurial spirit is admirable, it raises interesting anomalies if products considered inappropri-ate to show in an open clinic are advertised in the more intimate environ-ment of cyberspace. An important addition in this area of uncertainty was the conference "Interactive Health Communication for the Next Decade" the 1999 planning summit for health information developers held in Aptos, California in June 1999. Its principal sponsors were the Office of Health Promotion and Disease Prevention, the National Cancer Institute and the US Department of Health and Human Services. This conference drew from a publication by the Science Panel on Interactive Communication and Health as a resource. The deliberations and recommendations of the Science Panel on Interactive Communication and Health[70] are a major contribution to the debate of the evidence base for health care information to patients and the associated issues in deriving this information-based infrastructure.

DIRECT ACCESS OF PATIENTS TO TELEHEALTH SERVICES AND THE FUTURE OWNERSHIP OF PATIENT DATA

There are many issues still to be resolved in using telehealth in routine clin-ical practice:

+ Medicolegal issues
+ Medical licensure

- Reimbursement for services
- Appropriateness of use
- Data protection
- Bringing patients' clinical data together in a common format

While these issues are being discussed, there are patients who believe in the benefits of telehealth and are prepared to purchase telehealth services themselves. Using the Internet, people anywhere in the world can access advice on medical problems from a group of physicians with emergency room experience based in Boston. Patients with ischemic heart disease can now pay to have their heart rate, rhythm, and ECG monitored remotely.

An interesting aspect of these examples is the potential for conflict about who owns patient data. Physicians and health care organizations have previously taken a paternalistic approach to ownership of clinical data. Although patients can now see their records, worries about the security of medical records is a serious impediment to the future expansion of telehealth. In the United States the electronic patient record now makes it possible for some organizations to transmit records across distances to another institution when required in an emergency. In theory, a patient admitted to a hospital in New York could have his/her records transmitted electronically from Salt Lake City, Utah, and vice versa. The current reality is often different. Although this exchange is technically achievable, it is often practically impossible. There are barriers to hospitals sharing information in this way because of concerns about who owns the patient data, to which are attached medicolegal and financial concerns about sharing.

The Internet is a widely accessible network that health care organizations could use to help deliver services to patients. In the United States the Health Care Financing Administration (HCFA) has yet to report unequivocally its recommendations about issues related to the Internet and security of health care information. In the meantime the situation remains unclear. Will people with no access to health care because they have no insurance use Internet medical services as a provider of last resort? This may be a difficult area for legislation. Governments are finding this out in another area as they attempt to tax Internet services. Encryption of data solves data exchange on the Internet at one level of hierarchy, but the question of who owns the data remains an open question. Patients are beginning to lay claim to their clinical data as their own. How will this affect the question of data exchange in health care?

Interfacing between different data sources is a problem for the development of health information resources. A recent advance is Extensible Markup Language (XML). This promises to offer the same capacity to interface data sources that HTML has offered in linking graphic information. Exchanging data between different hospitals and physicians within and between countries is complicated by the different ways they store their medical history data. XML enables data sets to be exchanged by user-defined tags to mark and describe data. The resulting XML documents are built from elements defined by these custom tags.

THE FUTURE OF PATIENT PARTICIPATION IN HEALTH CARE AND TELEHEALTH

We are on the cusp of a huge wave of social change that is being generated by the information age in which we live. There promises to be more Internet shopping and more people working from home courtesy of computer links to their workplace. The city center department store and factory gave way to the local shopping mall and business park. Even these may prove to be intermediate social constructions on the way to ever more activity taking place from home. Health care may follow a similar pattern and be delivered directly into the home in a far higher percentage of situations. What this means for us as social animals enjoying "real" human contact remains to be seen. Opportunities and losses can be anticipated with all these changes. Currently, the loudest voices expressing opinions on what these changes mean for health care are coming from health care professionals, not patients. We have very little data about patient reactions to telehealth. Few telehealth studies include detailed consumer evaluations. However, one area where there are some preliminary data about using telehealth to support patients is that of providing health care to sick children in hospitals in the United States.

There are particular social challenges in caring for sick children in hospitals. These include keeping their morale high, providing social contact, preventing isolation, and giving them peer support. The hospital is very much an adult world into which children are placed and where they are relatively powerless over what happens to them. The work of the Starbright Foundation in Los Angeles has been an important contribution to advancing understanding of the needs of children in hospital and improving contribution to advancing understanding of the needs of children in hospital and improving the quality of their hospital experience. Preliminary work of the Starbright Foundation in association with Mount Sinai Medical Center in New York suggested telehealth interventions could promote recovery, shorten hospital stays, and decrease the amount of patient medication needed by children in hospital. From an initial pilot in 6 centers in the United States this project has now expanded to 40 centers. The work of the Starbright Foundation enables children to interact together between these centers in an

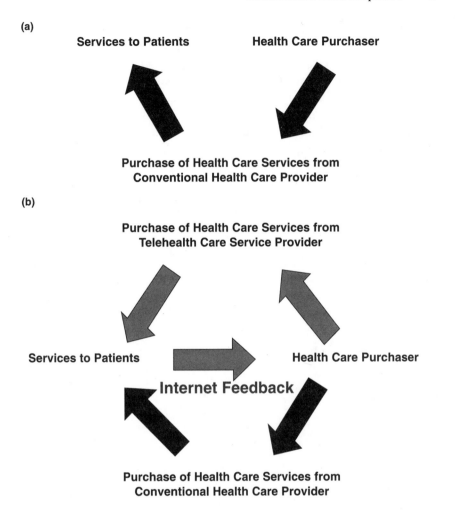

Figure 2.2 (a) Conventional health care purchasing and providing; (b) a new model of health care delivery with telehealth.

imaginative three-dimensional multi-media world. The children can use on-screen space to play together through the medium of real-time video conferencing, audio-linkage, typewritten text, chat rooms, and e-mail. It creates a network through which seriously ill children can develop a virtual community—Starbright World. Starbright World is a private and secure network through which children can also access the Internet and it ensures no inappropriate hot links are active. The work of the Starbright Foundation emphasizes the importance of the health care consumer in telehealth.

Published data from their work suggest direct benefits to the health care provider include reductions in pain intensity, pain aversiveness, and anxiety.[71]

So far, the future of telehealth frequently misses half of the equation standing to benefit from it—the patient perspective. Using telehealth to provide patients with the same information that doctors receive may radically change the dynamics of how health care is delivered in the future. It also may result in reduced costs and increased coverage, a magic formula so far eluding us. Figure 2.2 (see p. 45) illustrates the way in which telehealth may supplement conventional ways of delivering health care by providing a connection between patient and purchaser and also by offering the direct delivery of health care services to patients by telehealth providers.

3

Telehealth and Relationships with Physicians

Health care systems in Western industrialized countries such as the United States, United Kingdom, and Canada are now more preoccupied with treating chronic illnesses than with the acute life-threatening infectious diseases of the recent past. Because of this change, decisions made in health care are now usually about whether to treat, how to treat, when to treat, and how long to treat. Patients are realizing that there are risks as well as benefits to treatment and so demand more involvement in making any treatment decision of which they will bear the ultimate consequences. Telehealth offers an ideal tool to promote this sharing of information and help in managing patients with chronic diseases, especially in primary care. In doing this, telehealth changes aspects of the conventionally accepted roles of both patient and physician in the doctor–patient relationship. This chapter explores what these changes mean from the physician's perspective and suggests how relationships with physicians can be sensitively managed to help ensure telehealth programs are introduced successfully.

THE CHANGING ROLE OF PROFESSIONALS
IN THE INFORMATION AGE

As societies are moving from the industrial and postindustrial ages to the information age, we are seeing changes affecting the traditional professions of law, medicine, and architecture. In many ways the historical function of these three professions has been to act as specialized "knowledge keepers," requiring professional representation by bodies with purposes similar to those of the medieval guilds that protected aspects of commerce and trade in preindustrial society. We have seen how industrial mechanization changed the medieval guild system forever. Machines were able to replicate the work of traditional craftsmen faster, in greater volume, and at much lower cost. We may now be seeing the professions facing similar pressure to change because of recent advances in computing and information technology systems. Computer technology and networks are rapidly evolving from menial calculating machines to "knowledge machines" able to provide specialist information and expertise to people. In law, medicine, and architecture such knowledge machines are able to perform some of the tasks previously done by professionals and perform them faster, in greater volume, with higher accuracy, and at lower cost.

Central to the development of these knowledge machines are databases—tools to store, retain, correlate, and retrieve information digitally. With databases, the reservoirs of knowledge previously held by societies in books and journals requiring professional expertise to compile and disseminate are becoming freely available to anyone. The combination of databases and the Internet coupled with advances in data storage and data mining make repositories of knowledge available to the ordinary home that would have been unthinkable twenty years ago. The implications of this change for health care in general and telehealth in particular are enormous. Until 20 years ago the time taken for new knowledge to diffuse down into routine clinical practice in health care systems was painfully slow. It was common to find physicians who had practiced for a lifetime on a combination of their original medical school education, personal experience, and the occasional smattering of pharmaceutical literature. Inconsistencies in the knowledge base and level of practical expertise among physicians meant that the outcome of care for a patient could depend as much on the lottery of from which physician they sought treatment as much as from the effects of their disease. Intolerance with these variations in professional competency created inevitable pressure for the development of continuing medical education (CME) programs and the reaccreditation of physicians. Telehealth now offers us the possibility of placing expert systems on every physician's desktop. These expert systems will soon be able to give

- Treatment protocols for a range of common chronic conditions and statistical data on the outcomes patients can expect if treated using these.

+ Access to databases and bulletin boards giving on-line information on the latest treatments and how these may affect the prognosis of patients when used in the management of a particular disease or condition.
+ Access by videoconsultation and by remote analysis techniques (e.g., x-ray reporting) to particular experts who can give specialist advice in cases where there are doubts about the correct diagnosis or optimal treatment for a patient.

When this new package arrives on the physician's desk, it has the potential to change medicine as radically as industrial machines changed craft workshops over a century ago. We are likely to see dramatic changes in the doctor–patient relationship as a result. One possible scenario is that physicians will no longer need to maintain the appearance of being autonomous experts who know everything. Instead, they can concentrate their efforts on becoming sympathetic listeners and experts in supportive decision making, who help patients understand and then find solutions to the problems they present with. In this scenario the fact that a physician may admit to being unsure about what to do in a particular situation need not be a problem for doctor or patient. The likelihood is patients will adapt and find it normal and natural for a physician to ask for second opinions on-line and access information from a range of resources to help reach the "right" decision about treatment, based on the best available evidence. If this happens, patients will need to have this advice presented in ways to help them jointly decide with their physician what is the "right" treatment. Then it will become necessary for physicians to have the skills to help patients understand how to assess the evidence presented and use this to make decisions—decisions reflective of what the patient's preferences are rather than, as currently, the physician often instinctively making decisions on behalf of his/her patients.

We see other possible future scenarios for how physicians will adapt to these knowledge machines. In this respect health care has exact equivalents in the fields of law and architecture. In an information age the dilemma posed by the evolution of knowledge engines for the professions is that they threaten to reduce professional autonomy and cut monetary rewards in the future. In retrospect, the advantage of the factory and the reasons it triumphed over individual craftsmen were that it meant goods could be produced more cheaply and in greater quantities and then sold to a wider market. The need for individual craftsmen did not disappear as a result of industrialization; instead, they either catered to a different market or chose to work under different conditions. Inevitably, the personal autonomy of craftsmen changed. As we see these dramatic changes in the professional practice, the health care professions should ask themselves the following questions as they define strategies to cope with the information age:

- Are "information machines" cheaper and more efficient than a comparable professional for some aspects of their work?
- Is using technology cheaper and more efficient? If so, will health care professionals accommodate this change and so enable more people to access professional help more cheaply?
- Will patients as health care consumers choose to use new routes for obtaining health care advice and treatment instead of continuing to use traditional types of professional services?

These questions don't relate just to health care professionals. Consumers must inevitably play a decisive role in deciding the future because power and autonomy in society has moved to the consumer. Will consumers of health care choose to stay with the traditional model of the doctor–patient relationship, or will they exert pressure for change? Because physicians are not clear about what their patients want as consumers of health care, there is considerable anxiety on both sides. Telehealth is expanding rapidly in the area of giving information to patients. We believe that the future extent of the introduction of telehealth into health care delivery depends primarily on how well it integrates into the doctor–patient relationship. Although telehealth has important implications for other health care professionals, the changes are likely to be most acute in the doctor–patient relationship.

With the extent of change currently taking place, many physicians feel unsure about exactly how they should relate to their patients. This sense of isolation leaves them in a quandary. They feel unhappy with interference in the doctor–patient relationship and question the legitimacy of outside intrusions. The doctor–patient relationship is something most physicians still see as a private preserve, where any deficiencies should be dealt with in-house. This situation has the risk of denial and the real danger that sections of the medical community will become trapped like rabbits in the headlight beam of a car—unable to move and change position. This situation could be disastrous for physicians, patients, and health care systems alike. The ultimate strength of a health care system relates to the doctor–patient relationship and the duty of care that goes with it.

In the past the main emphasis in the training of physicians and other practitioners was to develop linear thinkers. Examination systems valued this ability. A challenge for medical education in the 21st century is the adaptation existing physicians and the preparation of those in training for a world where change is rapid and three-dimensional. Telehealth is a part of this same three-dimensional process of change affecting doctors and the doctor–patient relationship; things are constantly altering in time, space, and definition. Consequently, the effective introduction of telehealth programs into health care delivery systems requires an appraisal of the role of the physician in contemporary society. To understand how telehealth programs must adapt to physicians and physicians accommodate to telehealth systems requires the following considerations:

- A sense of the important fundamentals underpinning the doctor–patient relationship.
- Knowledge of the forces affecting the doctor–patient relationship and of why this relationship is currently under threat.
- The objectives of the doctor–patient relationship.
- Why doctors may feel threatened by the introduction of telehealth systems.
- How telehealth can help physicians meet their objectives in the doctor–patient relationship.

THE TRADITIONAL DOCTOR–PATIENT RELATIONSHIP AND HOW IT EVOLVED

There are no clearly defined contractual roles and responsibilities for the respective parties in the doctor–patient relationship. The respective roles of physician and patient originally emerged and have since adapted as part of human social evolution. From Aristotle's time, new physicians have trained in medicine as apprentices to practicing physicians. Student physicians learned how they, as physicians, related to patients through word of mouth and by emulating the behavior of their teachers. Throughout human history society and physicians have agreed upon guiding principles to establish the "proper" role of the doctor. These principles are generally available in society as codes of practice.

Hippocrates in ancient Greece codified the way physicians should behave. In doing this he emphasized the personal responsibility physicians have for their patients.[72] The paternalistic ethos of the Hippocratic code formed the ethical foundation for the subsequent development of Western allopathic medicine. This ethos had hardly changed by early part of the 20th century, when the role of the physician was neatly summarized by the following aphorism: "The secret of care of the patient is caring for the patient."[73]

As biomedical science advanced during the second half of the 20th century, medicine came to focus predominantly on disease. With this focus came an emphasis on the physicians ability to make a clear diagnosis in pathophysiological terms as the main objective of the medical consultation. In the 1960s the centrality of diagnostic certainty in the practice of medicine was illustrated by the following "call to stethoscope:"

> Diagnosis has two major objectives. One is to characterize the nature of the pathologic process in scientific and impersonal terms. The other is to evaluate the consequences of these processes in the individual patient. The first is the disease and the second is the illness.[74]

In terms of broad brush strokes over the course of 2500 years, the practice of medicine moved like a social tectonic plate away from simply caring for illness in people and took on the new orientation of making rational diagnoses and scientifically treating disease. In doing so the primary responsibility of physicians extended to include establishing the presence of disease and then assuming a duty of care for the patient, including a responsibility for treatment. Effects of this historical progression were not only to leave patients and other health care professionals with subordinate and passive roles. It also emphasized the unique importance of the doctor–patient relationship. Legislation and licensing powers further added to the new power base of physicians by making them powerful gatekeepers with autonomous control over what services patients could and should receive from a health care system. Inexorably, an unequal power relationship developed in Western allopathic health care systems, a relationship that would become problematical for doctors, patient, and society for three reasons:

- The doctor's duty of care to patients is often open-ended—what are the limits to diagnosis, treatment, and caring?
- The financial costs of diagnosis and treatment often are not factored in. Somebody has to pay—patient, taxpayer, or employer.
- Patients now say they want their own say in choices about their diagnosis and treatment, choices similar to those they have come to expect in other areas of our consumer-driven societies.

Medicine's centrality in the diagnosis and treatment of disease therefore created problems as well as benefits. The alignment of responsibility for diagnosis and treatment in one individual can make the potential costs of either infinite, whereas the resources available to meet them are strictly limited. Unfortunately, the biomedical model was never set up with boundaries to what clinical or financial constraints should guide physicians in practice. When health care was less technologically advanced and people's expectations of it were lower, there was no need. Eventually patients, employers, and governments have been forced to intervene. But how should these clinical and financial boundaries be set? The dislocation this is causing is one reason the doctor–patient relationship is under such strain from both inside and outside the relationship. This dynamic is of particular importance for telehealth. It is easy for a telehealth program to become mired in underlying frictions in the relationship between doctors and the health care systems in which they work. Before considering these wider aspects it is important to look in general terms at the doctor–patient relationship as it currently operates. Obviously, the relationship between any single patient and his/her single physician can lie within a hugely variable spectrum. This is a dynamic situation.

CURRENT CHALLENGES IN THE DOCTOR–PATIENT RELATIONSHIP

Even without added pressure from new developments such as telehealth, the traditional doctor–patient relationship faces challenges. Many physicians find it increasingly difficult to meet the growing expectations of their patients.[75] As a result, doctors often feel "out of tune" with what their patients want, so there is growing unease on both sides in the traditional framework of the doctor–patient relationship. Physicians are aware of a dissonance in what they and patients want from the relationship, so they look for new ways to relate to patients. Many doctors find this difficult. Until very recently, physician training did not include training in communication, conflict resolution, and negotiation skills. Physicians who have never needed to acquire these skills formally can find it hard to deal with patients who are now demanding greater autonomy, more information, and an increased say in any decisions made about the health care they receive. Ironically, as some patients reject the outmoded credo that asked them to believe that their "doctor knows best,"[76] others are seeking ever more reassurance and support from their doctors. Often physicians are inadequately trained to deal with these ambiguities or to provide this constant reassurance.

Physicians who were trained in a previous mold and cast as "helpful healers" whose role it was to decide what should be done to patients in their "best interest" find it hard when many patients now reject this model of medical practice and it is pejoratively referred to as paternalistic. Current pressure to change the doctor–patient relationship centers around an evolving concept of informed patients who take responsibility for deciding their own treatment from a range of possible choices. This concept removes the paternalism from the doctor–patient relationship and replaces it with a new consensual interaction. In this new model the doctor's role becomes one of friend, guide, counselor, and information giver to his/her patients. Telehealth fits well with this new model because it develops doctors as mentors and communicators. The role of the physician evolves to include educating patients and offering them evidence to support their choosing from among the available treatment options.

The External Environment: Managed Care

As well as inside the doctor–patient relationship, physicians face challenges from outside the relationship. Managed care as an organizational delivery system for health care is being cloned into various health care systems around the world. In its current form it threatens to further erode the traditional power and autonomy doctors have come to expect when practicing medicine. Managed care makes physicians accountable to management systems for any clinical and financial decisions they make on their patients' behalf. Data from clinical and financial databases are used to audit individual physicians' practices. These data are then compared with normative data derived from the practice of other comparable physicians and used as a tool to regulate how an individual physician should behave. Because of this, physicians see managed care as further removing the autonomy of choice that individual doctors have in making the "best" decisions they can for patients.[77,78] Managed care's primary concern has been to try to control the economic consequences of doctors' choices. It has not concerned itself with trying to iron out any inequalities in the power relationship between doctors and patients except when they directly affect the business of health care or explicitly harm patients. This does not mean managed care achieves the "right" result of empowering patients for the "wrong" reason. Far from it. Managed care may even create greater conflict for doctors in relating to patients. It can place doctors in situations where they have to act as patient advocates, yet at the same time work as entrepreneurs for a for-profit organization.[79]

Telehealth is an area where physicians must work with managed care organizations to ensure attempts at streamlining clinical practice take place with the safety of patients and practitioners in mind. Telehealth can support physicians, nurse practitioners, and physician's assistants to work in new roles, improving the access of patients to care based on clinical guidelines and protocols. A current climate of distrust exists about the underlying motives of managed care organizations felt by physicians and patients. This often makes physicians resist the changes in clinical practice necessary to embrace a new development such as telehealth. The seeming reluctance of physicians to accept telehealth as a way of delivering care contrasts with the readiness of patients to use telehealth as an information tool. It is important that physicians do not compromise their credibility in the doctor–patient relationship by using their time with patients to air their differences with new environments in which they work, such as telehealth. Patients' belief in the professional integrity of physicians is too important as a component of health care to be lost.

In many countries, including the United States, the United Kingdom, and Canada, there is a growing public malaise about the "health" of the health care systems because of changes patients perceive in the doctor–patient relationship. Although they may have some reservations, most people trust the competency of their own physicians but have less trust in the medical profession as a whole. Their main fears are about where health care systems seem inevitably headed—toward rising prices and reduced entitlements. This creates a general milieu of distrust, making many physicians feel trapped. They are constrained on one side by regulations and bureaucracy that restrict the level of care they can give to patients and on the other side by fears that these outside restrictions expose them to litigation from the patients they are desperately trying to care for. These social tensions put further strain on the doctor–patient relationship and add to the falling vote of public confidence in the quality of care delivered by their health care systems.[80]

Major Social Questions

Doctors and patients are constantly trying to form and sustain relationships amid the contradictions and ambiguities of the health care systems in which they must now meet. Major social questions about health care affect the relationship between doctors and patients, questions that doctors can't resolve either individually or within groups. These include the following:

- Is universal access to health care is a good thing? Is the dilemma not about providing health care but about who will pay? In the absence of properly funded universal health care, what constitutes a "safety net" service? If this is left to large hospitals to provide is this appropriate, and how should it be funded?
- If health care services no longer accept the physician's role in independently gauging the quality and appropriateness of care provided to patients, then what clinical outcome measures can replace clinical judgment? The move toward clinical outcomes questions the effectiveness of current practice and the benefits of technological advance, and it leads to anxieties about the cost, appropriateness, and quality of care.

What should stay and what should go in health care, and who should decide?

+ Why is it that the United States, United Kingdom, and Canada, with the most sophisticated health care technologies available, have sections of society with poor indices of health, such as perinatal mortality and life expectancy? What is the right balance of services among hospital care, primary care, and preventive services? How much should be spent on each?

+ How can government and purchasers of health and social care make distinctions between what is social care and what is health care? How can this be done equitably for populations and not cause ambiguity for professionals in the field?

Telehealth can help tackle some of the resource and allocation issues affecting wider health care systems in many countries facing these problems. Current public policy agendas make it difficult to introduce telehealth to address these problems. Government agencies in many countries are often facilitators of the development of an infrastructure, such as telehealth, for example, by grant programs but not by directly involving themselves in the process of delivering care. They are now seeing that they have two roles: (1) creating the right climate for market solutions to operate and (2) offering a safety net for people for whom the market cannot find solutions. The existing market signals associated with the doctor–patient relationship and telehealth are weak. This is because of cost containment and also because the cost improvements that telehealth has to offer health care systems are difficult to realize. The expenditure and revenue-saving possibilities in health care delivery systems often sit in different pockets of the same public purse. Savings from one pocket are not necessarily directly transferable to the other. In the private sector, physicians who help save costs by introducing new technology such as telehealth may see these savings lost into the wide corporate pot.

We see the early stages of creating telehealth networks as prime candidates for strategic planning and central direction from government. In the United States, government has taken the initiative in developing a strategy for a National Information Infrastructure (NII), including telehealth,[81] and has made considerable grant funding available to support this. The United Kingdom has no similar strategy.[82] Despite the levels of support, lack of coordination between central initiatives and an immature telehealth market often make telehealth programs difficult to introduce. As with other problems in health care delivery, the collective strains often appear first in the doctor–patient relationship.

In other areas of society, job descriptions and personnel specifications are used by organizations to reduce tension and strain in working relationships. Clear role definitions help arbitrate between what is expected of an individual and what the person can actually deliver within the organizational framework in which they work. In the United Kingdom where doctors in the NHS are more clearly seen as employees, medical staff have clear job descriptions for the first time. We believe telehealth programs must clearly outline the job descriptions and objectives for all practitioners, including doctors, and spell out the clinical and managerial tasks expected of them. Whether the telehealth program operates in a private or public setting, job descriptions can help with contracting as well as interpersonal relations. The current fragmentation of health care systems makes job descriptions particularly important for medicolegal reasons. In deriving these job descriptions it is helpful to have a clear idea of the objectives of the doctor–patient relationship.

OBJECTIVES OF THE DOCTOR–PATIENT RELATIONSHIP

In past situations, where health care interventions were mainly bed rest, nursing care, and isolation, loosely setting the objective of the physician as just to "care for the patient"[73] may have been sufficient. The expansion of medical science in the 1950s and 1960s introduced more therapeutic and surgical interventions, with risks as well as benefits. This expansion also opened up the doctor–patient relationship to scrutiny from a wider social perspective. Studies by sociologists, psychiatrists, psychologists, educators, and doctors now offer a much greater breadth of understanding of the objectives in the doctor–patient relationship. Research suggests that physicians should manage the doctor–patient consultation to achieve three basic outcomes:[83]

- ◆ Determine the nature of the patient's problem and make a diagnosis.
- ◆ Develop and then maintain or conclude a therapeutic relationship.
- ◆ Include patient education in the treatment plan.

We believe physicians conducting telehealth consultations in routine clinical practice should find ways of incorporating these three basic functions into their consultations. Physicians usually learn clinical methods, including history taking, examination, making diagnoses, and prescribing treatments, by a system of rote learning. This teaching method has not traditionally considered the building of relationships with patients as having equivalent importance to finding disease. Telehealth requires physicians to move outside the disease-based approach of the clinical method and define exactly what kind of relationship they are trying to build with a patient. We often find in working with physicians to introduce telehealth that it is the first time many have considered fundamental issues related to solving patients' problems.

Telehealth As a Clinical Tool to Determine the Nature of Patients' Problems and Help in Making a Diagnosis

Most patients have tried self-medication and discussing their health problems with a family member or friends before they eventually resort to visiting a doctor for help.[84] Telehealth could play a major role at this initial stage of helping people decide whether or not to see a doctor. Some patients hesitate about going to visit their doctor when they unquestionably need care, and others make unnecessary appointments to see doctors. Printed information about self-care can reduce physician visits to patients by 17% and reduce patient visits to doctors for minor illnesses by 35%.[85] These findings form the basis for "demand management"[86] in health care. This and similar programs use telephone triage to reduce the demand levels of patients for health care services or channel them efficiently into the most appropriate form of care. Telehealth activity, particularly through the Internet, is set to play an important role in educating people about self-help and about how they can access health care appropriate to their needs. It also can provide health promotion and disease prevention programs. The experience of triage systems is that this is most effectively done by using clear guidelines and protocols for care.

Patients feel that their problems have been adequately assessed when they see a doctor if they understand the following from the consultation:

+ What has caused their problems and symptoms.
+ What will happen to their health as a consequence of these problems and symptoms—both treated and untreated.

In traditional face-to-face consultations, patients are typically able to convey only one quarter to one third of their concerns to a physician.[87] This is partly because of time constraints and partly because of the physician's traditional focus on confirming or excluding disease. Once the consultation begins, physicians typically interrupt the patients within 18 seconds of first asking them to describe their concerns.[88] Despite what at first seem formidable communication constraints, doctors make a diagnosis from the patient's history in 60%–80% of cases.[89–91] Figures 3.1 and 3.2 show ways in which telehealth can be used in determining the problem and making a diagnosis.

The inability to examine a patient directly is frequently raised as a criticism of telehealth's capacity to discover patients' problems and make a correct clinical diagnosis. The fact that face-to-face consultations the correct clinical diagnosis is usually made in 60%–80% of cases from the clinical history alone suggests that telehealth should be able to make a correct diagnosis in the majority of cases as long as a detailed clinical history is taken. But how good is telehealth at interpreting physical signs and investigations? Clinical research comparing telehealth with conventional methods of clinical examination and interpreting investigations suggests that telehealth is a reliable way of making clinical diagnosis remotely.

Remote interpretation of physical signs and clinical investigations using telehealth is classifiable into three basic patterns, depending on whether or not additional technology is used and if so what type of technology is employed.[92] *Pattern 1* emerges when a remote stethoscope and telemedicine camera is used. This pattern is associated with diagnostic errors when the clinician was not fully trained in the use of these techniques. *Pattern 2* occurs when a remote examiner performs a physical examination and will then need to learn new skills to become competent in clinical diagnosis. In *pattern 3*, information is transferred digitally (e.g., ultrasound and ECG), and the diagnostic accuracy is usually the same as when the investigations are interpreted conventionally.

This analysis of diagnostic patterns suggests that telehealth is a reliable method of finding out about patients' problems and then making an accurate clinical diagnosis. It also suggests that the skills of conventional physical examination and interpretation of investigations are not directly transferable to the telehealth situation. Clinicians require training in the examination

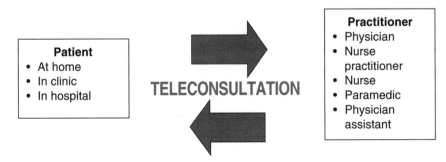

Figure 3.1   Real-time video conferencing between a practitioner and a patient or between a practitioner and patient and another specialist practitioner.

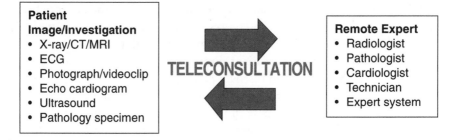

Figure 3.2   Store-and-forward techniques where pictures, x-rays, and other diagnostic images are sent for review by specialist experts.

techniques of telehealth. If they are trained, they can achieve comparable results to conventional examination techniques. The three patterns of skill acquisition in telehealth consultation are shown in Figure 3.3.

The diagnostic accuracy of telehealth consultations does not have to be 100% equivalent to conventional methods of clinical practice to make telehealth a workable proposition. If a telehealth application is consistently reliable in a sufficient percentage of cases and is of high quality and lower cost, it can safely replace some, but not all, elements of conventional clinical practice. In the rest of clinical situations, where telehealth is uncertain, then the default position of conventional practice applies. A good example of this is the use of telehealth by nurse practitioners in minor treatment centers.[93]

The conventional practice of medicine is usually based on arriving at diagnostic certainty. A physician tries to make a definitive diagnosis as a result of being certain of the clinical history, clinical examination, and the results of the diagnostic tests relating to a particular patient. In contrast, telehealth is often a useful tool in situations of clinical uncertainty. For example, in rural and remote areas clinicians often need help in exploring diagnostic uncertainty and then deciding whether a patient should be transferred to a specialist center for further treatment. When the clinical condition of patients is unstable, their transfer by ambulance to a specialist center may involve considerable risks and costs. In such situations the advantage of telehealth is that it can "virtually" transfer a specialist expert to assess the patient at the remote site instead of transferring the patient with its attendant risks.

A good example of where this can help is in managing patients with severe head injuries. Patients with head injuries from road traffic accidents often have other associated injuries to their chest, neck, abdomen, and limbs. The main reason for transferring the patient to a specialist center

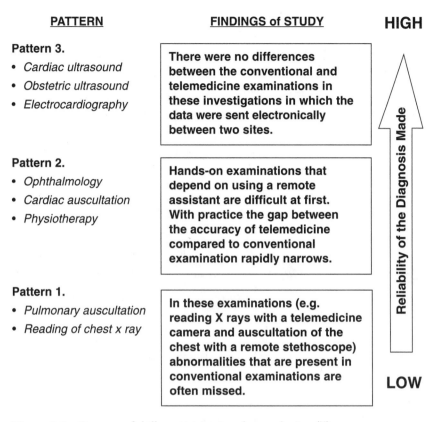

Figure 3.3   Patterns of skill acquisition in teleconsultation.[92]

(e.g., neurosurgical center) is to treat a traumatic blood clot compressing the brain, should one be present, and to manage primary brain injuries. By remote assessment of the patient and CT scan an unnecessary transfer of an unstable patient can be avoided, or the rapid transfer of a patient at serious risk can be expedited. When people compare telehealth with conventional treatment of patients, they often focus on the lack of absolute certainty with telehealth and reject its use. In doing so they miss the point. The very strength of telehealth is usually in its capacity to deal with uncertainty. Figure 3.4 shows diagrammatically how the reduction in diagnostic uncertainty applies when using telehealth.

An area of controversy where further clarification is needed in telehealth is in using a remote telemedicine camera to assess x-rays. Telemedicine cameras are a valuable adjunct in the emergency treatment of patients when the primary clinician is unsure of the most appropriate step to take;[93] however, the use of telemedicine cameras to interpret x-rays can result in

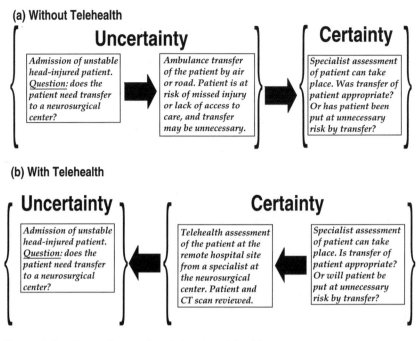

Figure 3.4   Uncertainty and certainty in telehealth.

abnormalities on chest x-rays being missed such as when x-rays are sent for review to a physician in a pulmonary clinic.[92] The American College of Radiology (ACR) and the National Electrical Manufacturers Association (NEMA) have jointly set technical standards to define the resolution requirements of teleradiology systems.[94,95] In some situations access to somebody with greater knowledge in the management of the patient's problem may outweigh the imperfections in the resolution of transmitted images associated with using an ordinary telemedicine camera to view the x-rays. Weighing the risks and benefits of using a telemedicine camera not meeting professional standards involves complex medicolegal and professional considerations. Using a telemedicine camera for diagnosis in telehealth programs should be undertaken with caution and should take place only in the context of agreed-on clinical protocols, where all clinicians involved share collective responsibility.

Accuracy of diagnosis is not only important to the doctor and patient for medicolegal reasons. It is also important to telehealth programs for reimbursement. When patients are discharged, the medical diagnosis is used to decide the level of reimbursement/cost capture in conventional treatment situations. For this same reason it is important telehealth consultations have a diagnostic label attached to them. The labels used for clinical diagnosis by practitioners vary. Common forms of diagnostic classification for coding purposes are shown in Table 3.1. The importance of the diagnosis is also one determinant of the necessity or otherwise of the clinician's being involved in the therapeutic relationship with the patient at various stages in telehealth.

Telehealth As a Tool to Develop, Maintain, and Conclude a Therapeutic Doctor–Patient Relationship

After a physician makes a working diagnosis, the doctor–patient relationship either continues as a therapeutic relationship or concludes with no further need for the doctor to see the patient again. One consultation may be all that is required if any of the following conditions applies:

- Doctor and patient are both satisfied and agree with the course of action.
- The patient is unsatisfied and wants to seek help elsewhere.
- The doctor feels there is no more she/he can offer.

Often the decision about whether to continue or to conclude the therapeutic relationship cannot be made at once because additional data are needed to make a diagnosis. Current models for delivering health care can make this into a protracted process, as shown in Figure 3.5.

Figure 3.6 shows how teleconsultation can save weeks or months in a primary care referral to a specialist physician. Telehealth achieves this by removing the delays in exchanging letters and scheduling appointments. A three-way consultation among a patient's primary care doctor, a specialist physician, and the patient reduces the communication delay, and all the parties involved can then be clear about the decision they eventually make together. Decisions about whether the therapeutic relationship should continue can be made sooner, with the advantages of less worry for the patient and less disruption to his/her family/work life. For the physician who faces

Table 3.1   Common Classification Systems for Reimbursement

- The International Classification of Disease (ICD-9)
- Diagnostic Related Groups (DRGs)
- Resource Based Relative Value System (RBRVS)
- Reed Classification (UK)
- Snowmed
- DSM-3 (psychiatry)

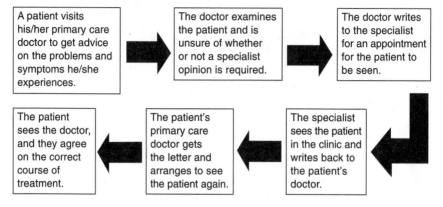

Figure 3.5   Delays resulting from conventional consultation methods.

the problem of the ever expanding scope of medical practice and ever multi-plying treatment options, telehealth makes it easier to get up-to-date advice and guidance for patients.

If a therapeutic relationship is to be ongoing, a physician must decide, regardless of whether she/he uses conventional practice or telehealth, what her/his role is in the patient's care. Is she/he a primary care physician, a specialist, or a temporary consultant to the patient? Telehealth makes any one of these roles possible. Not only medical considerations influence what type of doctor–patient relationship exists and whether it continues. Emotional,[96] cultural,[97] social,[98] and behavioral[99] factors are equally as important as the treatment offered in deciding whether a doctor–patient relationship remains ongoing. Consequently, telehealth programs must decide exactly what relationships they are trying to create between practitioners and patients. Because there are no clear data available, the effect of nontechnical aspects (e.g., emotion, culture, and behavior) on managing telehealth consultations is unclear.

Because so much emphasis is placed on the biomedical aspects of diagnosing and treating disease, the beneficial effect of just seeing a doctor is often forgotten. Just meeting the doctor and discussing a problem has a marked therapeutic effect.[100] Doctors should consciously try to integrate this therapeutic effect into the clinical consultation and use it to initiate new methods of dialogue between patients and themselves,[75] bringing the concept of shared decision making between doctor and patient into the consultation and letting the doctor empathize with the patient. There are not yet data to show whether the telehealth consultation has the same benefits. It may be that vital nonverbal cues are lost when using a camera for remote

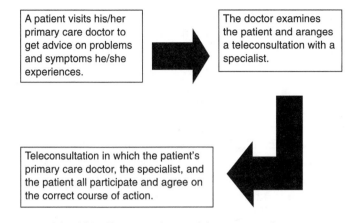

Figure 3.6   Telehealth's effect on reducing delays in consultation.

consultation. Research is needed in this as in other areas of doctor–patient interaction in telehealth.

The balance of power in the doctor–patient relationship has long favored the doctor, yet patients learn to influence the direction of the consultation to their advantage. Patients develop strategies, including presentation of emotional and social distress, to get around the biomedical approach.[101] Physicians are action-oriented and have strong incentives to intervene and treat symptoms. Patients do not always follow the treatment recommendations suggested. If patients fail to attend follow-up appointments or to take medication prescribed for them, they are described as noncompliant (a term which is being replaced by "nonadherent") with the treatment. In some situations using the label "noncompliant" reinforces the sense of medical paternalism of the doctor–patient relationship. Is noncompliance the physician's need to take control in the relationship? It could equally well be asked whether it is the patient or doctor who is noncompliant.[102] We are seeing interesting instances in telepsychiatry where patients who are anxious, uncooperative, and noncompliant in the conventional consultation are calmer in the teleconsultation. When asked why, their answer is "because [they] have the power to switch off the monitor and end the consultation," a power that, interestingly, they very seldom exercise.

A current dilemma for telehealth in maintaining the therapeutic relationship is how to share the patient case record between remote and referring physician in the consultation in most health care organizations. Systems integration of telehealth technology and patient information systems has not yet progressed to the stage where patient records and clinical investigations are easily shared between the two systems. This presents most difficulty when using interactive video systems for telehealth consultations and is usually easier in store-and-forward systems. The systems integration to accomplish this data interface will come in the near future. In the meantime it is sometimes a source of confusion and clinical risk.

Ending the Doctor–Patient Relationship

Inevitably, the doctor–patient relationship ends at some defined point in time. Patients can react to this with a sense of loss.[103] This sense of loss may result from breaking the previous dependency induced by the traditional doctor–patient interaction,[104] or it may be just the normal human process of saying good-bye to a friend.[105] Whatever the reason, when the therapeutic relationship is terminated, patients may show a variety of responses, as shown in Table 3.2.

Medical reluctance to end their therapeutic relationships with patients can arise when physicians have a "need to be needed" and fear they will hurt a dependent patient's feelings. Physicians can make the ending of the doctor–patient relationship easier by properly defining the relationship at the beginning.[106] The process of transition for patients is easier if they are informed at the end of the relationship about their future prognosis and if any plans for the transfer of care are clearly stated. Here are important lessons for telehealth programs. They must ensure teleconsultations fit into an overall plan of patient management, one that patients understand and accept. If not, these loose ends will need picking up in further traditional face-to-face consultations, and this will reduce the competitive advantage of the telehealth program by increasing costs. Patients are familiar with a one-to-one relationship with their physician. Telehealth means patients may share two clinicians simultaneously—a referring clinician and a remote physician. The role of the referring physician may be to share the care with a remote physician who acts as a purely technical expert. The referring physician also may need to take on the role of the patient advocate. In these situations of divided clinical responsibilities for telehealth it is important to make sure that patients are aware of when a therapeutic relationship has finished and who is responsible for undertaking any care in the future.

Patient Education

Physicians often miss the opportunity to provide patients with enough information in traditional consultations.[107,108] Patients must have adequate information if they are to fully participate in decisions about their care. Traditionally, health care information was exclusively the possession of health care professionals, particularly doctors. Much of a physician's professional

Table 3.2   Responses of Patients to Ending the Doctor–Patient Relationship

- Anger
- Noncompliance with a new physician
- A flare-up of the original symptoms
- Sadness
- Anxiety

power rested on being the guardian of health information from sources such as scientific journals and being the gatekeeper to services patients could receive. The situation is now changing. Literature, television, videos, and the Internet provide patients with an abundance of information about health care. Unfortunately, drawing on these rich sources of information does not necessarily help the drive toward equality in the doctor–patient relationship. How should the sources of information that telehealth makes available to doctor and patient be incorporated productively into the doctor–patient interaction? Patients who come to see their physician with seven pages of information from the Internet when there are only 15 minutes of consultation time available create a problem. How can physicians read and assimilate information from a wide variety of sources and then diagnose, advise, and treat in the time allotted to them? Information management in health care is crucial for the future. The physician's role is not to be the guardian of the information but to help patients understand information and use this to inform their choices.

In the realm of patient education, telehealth has an amazing opportunity to help in disseminating information to patients and then help them participate in decisions about their health. Realizing these benefits requires a clear vision of what information to provide to patients and of how to manage the process of information giving. As information consumers brought up in a television age, we expect our information edited, produced, and well presented. If telehealth is to succeed by using these media, it must emulate the standards we now expect in other areas of our lives.

THE DOCTOR–PATIENT RELATIONSHIP AND TELEHEALTH

Telehealth projects can either replicate the current model of the doctor–patient relationship or find a way to use the technology to offer new solutions and define new ways for doctors and patients to interact. In chapter 4 we view the teleconsultation as one way to resolve some of the challenges we have described in delivering health care services in the 21st century. There are no magic solutions, only trade-offs to make among the quality, cost, and access to health care services for populations. Finding where these trade-offs are possible involves working collaboratively with physicians and other practitioners. Good working relationships with doctors are vital to the future of telehealth programs.

WHY IS THE DOCTOR–PATIENT RELATIONSHIP IN TELEHEALTH AN ISSUE FOR DOCTORS?

When telehealth is used to provide health care services, there is some degree of physical separation of doctor from patient.[109] Physical separation of patients from their doctors lies behind much of the medical concern about telemedicine,[110] concern based on the strong belief that the traditional doctor–patient consultation is the gold standard to achieve in health care.[78] In reality, are teleconsultations inferior to face-to-face consultations with doctors? Are patients deprived when they don't have a direct face-to-face interaction with their doctor? We have very little objective data to draw on with which to give any ruling on these questions. In the absence of evidence to answer these questions, telehealth is often presumed guilty and summarily rejected. This rejection is despite the evidence that the traditional doctor–patient relationship has its own failings and that we need to find a new way to interact with patients, a way in which we believe telehealth will have a major part to play.

4

Using Telehealth to Make Health Care Transactions

A telehealth program's success ultimately depends on clinicians and patients using it for routine health care delivery. No matter how sophisticated the technology or how elaborate the clinical processes involved in telehealth, if these cannot translate into an adequate demand for teleconsultation, then the program is likely to fail. The health care consultation is often thought of simplistically as just a clinical encounter between a patient and practitioner, whereas in reality it is a much more involved process. Complex interactions take place behind the scenes to make a consultation possible. These processes include medicolegal considerations, managing clinical risk, and ensuring that adequate payment is received for the services provided. Telehealth programs are managing very sophisticated clinical encounters. This chapter considers current uses for telehealth and the support mechanisms to be managed effectively in consolidating the teleconsultation into a commercial health care transaction,[111] one that will provide the revenue on which the future of telehealth so crucially depends.

WHAT AREAS OF HEALTH CARE ARE SUITABLE FOR TELEHEALTH?

Microprocessors are a ubiquitous part of our everyday lives and have a vast untapped potential for changing the way health care services are delivered.

The health care industry is labor-intensive and still relies heavily on paper-based methods of communication. In almost every part of health care there is plenty of scope for information technology to support people and paper processes and so improve communication. As data networks are developed further among different sectors of the health care market, the opportunities for introducing telehealth will continually expand. In 1997 the US Federal Communications Commission Advisory Committee on Telecommunications sought to expand the provision of telemedicine in rural areas of America and looked for opportunities for developing telemedicine networks. As part of this process the committee described what they called a market basket of telemedicine applications. The market basket contained a range of telehealth activities that they envisioned could flourish if an adequate network infrastructure was present to support them at an economic price. This market basket for telehealth transactions is shown in Table 4.1. The thematic link among these various telehealth applications is delivering health care in situations where the giver and recipient of information are physically separated. Instead of having a direct physical connection the parties are linked by the transmission of sound, vision, image, or printout. Links utilizing the range of information technology are shown in Table 4.2.

The identity of the sender and receiver of health care services in telehealth varies according to the nature of the information/advice exchanged and other associated factors, such as geographical location and urgency of medical condition. Given the right infrastructure and acceptance by clinicians and patients, telehealth transactions could be developed to offer services throughout the health care delivery system.

WHAT IS A TELEHEALTH TRANSACTION?

We use the term "telehealth transaction" for particular telehealth applications in which the clinical, medicolegal, technical, contractual, and business aspects of telehealth all interface. This makes a telehealth transaction into a coalescence of purpose requiring the active management of the operational considerations listed in Table 4.3. One of the main lessons health care organizations are learning from successful sections of the business community is the importance of adopting a customer focus in the services they provide. Ultimately, the customers of a telehealth program are the practitioner and the patient who teleconsult. No matter how much is spent, no matter how sophisticated the equipment, if patient and practitioner do not buy into the process and teleconsult, a telehealth program cannot survive in the long term. Winning the enthusiastic buy-in of practitioner and patient is the

Table 4.1   A Market Basket of Telehealth Applications

- Health care to health care provider consultation—physician and non-physician health care providers (nurses, physician assistants, etc.) in hospitals and clinics consulting (includes triage) professionals in other locations and the transmission of data and medical images such as x-rays;
- Health care provider to patient consultation—patients in hospitals and clinics examining/counseling in a multimedia format depending on the need by physicians/ specialists and non-physicians (e.g., dieticians, occupational therapists, physical therapists, nurse specialists in clinical areas such as diabetes and mental health etc.) in medical centers for consultation and triage utilizing a variety of examination devices such as electronic stethoscopes, ophthalmoscopes, otoscopes, EKGs, etc;
- Physicians and other healthcare professionals and providers participating in continuing medical education programs;
- Healthcare providers having access to the most current medical information through the Internet;
- Emergency departments able to get 24 hour a day support (includes triage) from on-call physicians/specialists either at urban centers or at a local physicians office;
- A comprehensive set of specialty services such as radiology, dermatology, selected cardiology, pathology, obstetrics (fetal monitoring), pediatric, mental health/psychiatric should be enabled as a result of the capacity to transmit high speed data and high quality images to urban medical centers;
- Emergency departments and trauma centers in urban areas should be able to interact with paramedics directly at the scene in case of emergencies in most areas. Helicopters and ambulances transmitting real-time information on vital signs such as temperature, blood pressure, EKG, etc. to emergency departments or trauma centers in urban areas.[111a]

cornerstone on which the rest of the telehealth transaction depends. The preeminent telehealth programs of the future will be those that actively manage the telehealth transaction to ensure that it succeeds.

THE OPERATIONAL MANAGEMENT OF TELEHEALTH TRANSACTIONS

Many telehealth programs and companies are selling products to their health care customers based on the promise of teleconsultation's being cheaper and more convenient than conventional practice. These promises become empty when the telehealth equipment is delivered without also providing robust and worked-through models for how telehealth transactions will deliver this promised convenience and cost saving. The operational management issues for health care services adopting telehealth are shown in Table 4.4.

Table 4.2   Common Technologies for Telehealth

+ Telephone
+ Facsimile
+ Digital or analog land lines as data links
+ Satellite data linkage systems
+ Video-conferencing

Ensuring that Telehealth Fits into the
Existing Patterns of Care Delivery

If telehealth is substituted for a conventional system of providing health care services, it does not necessarily follow that the subsequent process of delivering health will work effectively. A simple example of this is trying to augment an existing dermatology service to outlying remote rural areas with a teledermatology system. Advantages of teledermatology are that it removes the unnecessary travel time of the dermatologist and the long waiting times of patients for office appointments. With the telehealth solution, primary care physicians or nurse practitioners can initially see the patient instead. Practitioners can then use the dermatology service to consult when they have doubts about a diagnosis. However, if the primary care physicians or nurse practitioners are unable to perform skin biopsies in place of the dermatologist and biopsies are a necessary part of the service, fixing the problem may require

+ Training the primary care physicians or nurse practitioners in skin biopsy.
+ Traveling long distances to the dermatologist.
+ Reinstituting the dermatologist's visits.
+ Abandoning the teledermatology service and reverting to the previous arrangement.

A more complex example of how a new telehealth service must interface with any existing service is providing a telepsychiatry service to an under-

Table 4.3   Considerations in Telehealth Transactions

+ The clinical rationale for teleconsulting
+ The practitioner–patient relationship
+ Risk management to reduce the possibility of harm to patients and subsequent litigation against the program
+ Choices of what technology is appropriate for the purpose proposed

Table 4.4   Operational Issues in Telehealth Transactions

* Ensuring that telehealth fits into the existing pattern of care delivery
* Scheduling of patients
* Reporting mechanisms and record keeping
* Storage of images
* Security issues
* Measurement of quality
* Comfort, convenience, and location
* Backup and fail-safe procedures
* Training of practitioners
* Education of patients

served remote rural area without psychiatrists. Part of the standard workup of most psychiatric patients is to exclude organic brain lesions (e.g., brain tumors, stroke, and hydrocephalus). This workup may call for a routine CT scan and/or MRI scan. Having first set up the telepsychiatry service, the health care purchaser may then need to cover the additional costs of the specialist investigations without which the psychiatrists cannot practice.

These examples emphasize how important it is to check whether any new process of care actually works before trying to replace an existing health care delivery system with a new telehealth solution. Figure 4.1 illustrates a conventional treatment process with an intact process of care. Figure 4.2 illustrates the effect of a proposed telehealth service introduced without first checking to see if the process of care remains intact. Figure 4.3 illustrates diagrammatically how processes of delivering care may require adapting to work with telehealth.

Scheduling Patients

It frequently seems a trite detail and is passed over in dealing with other immediate priorities, but telehealth systems often neglect to ensure that an adequate mechanism exists for their health care clients to use for scheduling consultations between the patients and practitioners who will use the new system. This is analogous to trying to sell trains to a railway system without a timetabling system and then wondering why the market for trains does not immediately take off. We have seen state-of-the-art telemedicine systems, with hundreds of thousands of dollars of investment, routinely scheduling patients to teleconsult with a specialist by telephoning a part-time secretary, who sends back appointment lists by conventional mail—and then letters are sent out to patients. Generally, there are three types of scheduling requirement for telehealth; these are shown in Table 4.5.

Table 4.5   Scheduling Arrangements for Telehealth Services

* Urgent consultation/immediate access
* Booked appointment
* Store and forward

Many telehealth networks are not yet advanced enough to offer immediate on-line teleconsultation advice unless they link to a constantly staffed facility such as an emergency room or an urgent x-ray reporting room. Immediate on-line access works in these situations because of redundancy in the conventional health care delivery arrangements that allow urgent teleconsultations to take place. The emergency room physician and the urgent reporting radiologist are already on site. The marginal cost and marginal effort of providing a telehealth service in this way is often small. If a telehealth service such as this becomes successful, the costs may suddenly escalate disproportionately when the volume of demand for the service means that extra members of staff must be employed to run it. This ad hoc system for immediate teleconsultation has the drawback that it may be able to take only one urgent teleconsultation at a time. Another way of offering urgent telehealth appointments is to use a pager or cellular telephone to connect to designated practitioners on an on-call rotation.

A booked appointment system is the route taken by most telehealth systems for offering routine real-time teleconsultation services. This operational requirement of this system closely follows an existing face-to-face outpatient clinic arrangement. The patient usually visits a remote consultation clinic in a primary care facility and consults with a practitioner (usually a doctor) who arranges to connect him/her to a distant outpatient clinic or office. The doctors offering the service change a proportion of their conventional consulting time to become scheduled teleconsultation time.

Store-and-forward telehealth involves taking and storing pictures (dermatology, ophthalmology, etc.) or images (x-ray, ultrasound, etc.) at the remote site and sending these for reporting. This system needs scheduling arrangements to enable those sending images to know when they can be reported.

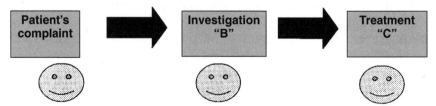

Figure 4.1   Conventional treatment with an intact process of care.

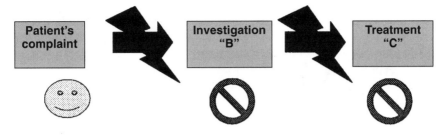

Figure 4.2   Proposed telehealth treatment without checking the integrity of process of care.

It also requires an audit trail to ensure that the dispatch and receipt of images is verified; any lost images, pictures, or reports can then be traced. Although using secretaries or clinic clerks to schedule appointments for telehealth consultations or to check on store-and-forward investigations can be efficient, we believe it is reminiscent of driving in the early 20th century, when having a person with a red flag walking in front of a motorcar was necessary. This is poor advertising for a telehealth system. It is usually only a small additional cost to a telehealth system to have a built-in scheduling system to help manage the work flow and reduce administrative costs. Figures 4.4 to 4.6 illustrate different ways of scheduling telehealth transactions in current use by operational telehealth services.

Reporting Mechanisms and Record Keeping in Telehealth

Consultations and investigations are performed in health care because they add to the sum total of knowledge about a patient's condition/disease and help

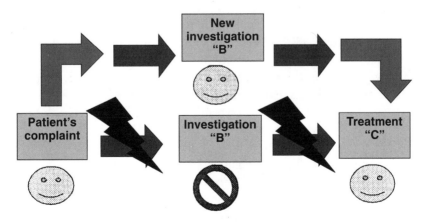

Figure 4.3   A proposed telehealth treatment with an intact process of care.

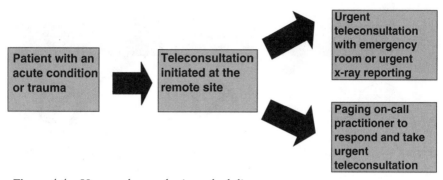

Figure 4.4   Urgent teleconsultation scheduling.

decide what, if any, future actions are needed. These consultations and investigations do not take place in isolation. They fit into wider processes of care for preventing ill health, treating disease, and palliating symptoms. Feedback mechanisms convey the results of any consultations and investigations back to patients and other practitioners so that decisions about care can be made. The results of these health care consultations and of investigations such as x-ray, ultrasound, and ECG are then filed and available in the patients' records. Such processes formally record how and why treatment choices are offered to patients. The purpose of keeping records is to allow other practitioners to understand the rationale for the management of each patient's condition and to form a lasting medicolegal record.

Telehealth consultations and investigations do not always fit into preexisting processes for reporting results and keeping records. Telehealth projects with only a small number of consultations to manage can usually work out a "one off" mechanism to integrate reporting and record keeping. This is more difficult with larger operational health care delivery services that rely on telehealth. Health care providers' information systems rarely have the capacity to electronically link and integrate patient records. Even if records can be linked and integrated, in many countries the legality of keeping electronic records in health care in place of traditional paper records is not yet clearly established. Issues that are still to be resolved in telehealth include (1) who keeps the clinical records? (2) where should the clinical records for telehealth be kept? (3) what data should they contain? These issues are illustrated by the example of using telehealth to provide remote advice for patients with chest disease, as shown in Figure 4.7.

When the patient is examined at the remote clinic site, a history, physical examination, and x-ray are all performed. The details of these are recorded in the patient's clinical record. What, if any, of this clinical record can then be transmitted to the specialist center in advance of the teleconsultation? If

Remote Clinic Site

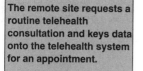

The remote site requests a routine telehealth consultation and keys data onto the telehealth system for an appointment.

Details of the appointment scheduled and displayed on the telehealth system.

Specialist Center

Request from remote site received and available clinic times displayed for selection of date, time, and specialty.

Remote site chooses the time, date, and specialty and books appointment.

Figure 4.5   Routine teleconsultation scheduling.

the patient is not already known to them, does the specialist center treat the referred patient as a new patient and open its own set of clinical notes? Does the specialist send a written record of the consultation to the remote site? What is the process for establishing an audit trail for the chest x-ray and ensuring that a report gets back to the remote site? These are important aspects of the consultation that must be integrated into the care delivery process.

The integration of this information is easier when the remote site and specialist center are both within the same organization and sharing a common information system. These problems of information integration will eventually be resolved when projects aimed at fully integrating patient records with other clinical systems finally deliver a robust product. In the meantime, interfacing a telehealth program with existing systems for recording and transmitting patient information is a major challenge that operational telehealth programs face when trying to deliver routine health care services in both the United States and the United Kingdom. It is also a source of considerable frustration to busy clinicians working in environments where time constraints exist.

Digital Storage of Images in Telehealth

A great potential benefit to using telehealth systems for imaging services is that images can be stored on digital systems.[112] Digital storage systems can be used for x-ray images, CT, MRI, ultrasound, ECG, video, and photographs. Some logistical considerations to take into account when investigating how feasible digital storage systems are for an organization are illustrated by examining issues involved in storing x-ray images digitally.

Conventional methods of storing and manually retrieving x-ray and ultrasound images are a labor-intensive and expensive undertaking. The replacement of x-ray films with digital images stored on optical disks makes

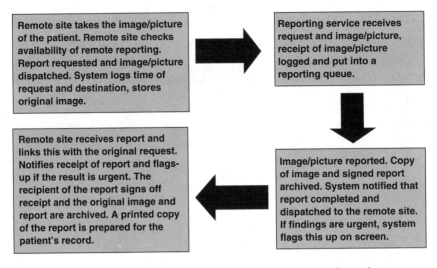

Figure 4.6   Store-and-forward consultation scheduling and audit trail.

logical sense in this context but does not automatically mean a practicable business case can be developed for a digital radiology storage system to accompany a teleradiology service. Digital teleradiology systems can save on the costs of storage space for x-ray films, clerical support to file x-ray films, and the purchase of x-ray films. If the volumes of x-ray images taken in a clinic are high enough, these savings may make a major contribution to the business case for investing in a teleradiology system that includes a digital image storage system; however, these direct costs are not the only considerations. X-ray films have other advantages when considered in the wider process of delivering clinical care. These advantages may override the purely radiographic considerations. X-ray films are portable and are easily transported around a clinic or hospital for viewing with the patient or with other practitioners. If patients are transferred to another hospital, x-ray films can be readily copied and sent along with them in an envelope. The legal status of x-rays films is clearly established; in many countries the legality of using digitally stored images as medical evidence instead of conventional x-ray films remains unresolved.

For a teleradiology system to offer physicians the same functionality in viewing x-ray images in clinics and on wards that conventional x-ray films offer requires a distributed digital information network onto which these images can be distributed. Factoring the additional costs of the network and display monitors with the required resolution to view the x-rays can make the costs of a digital image storage and retrieval system for teleradiology

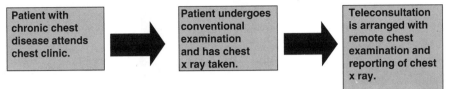

Figure 4.7   Reporting and record keeping in a telehealth clinic.

prohibitively expensive. Instead of converting to a fully digital teleradiology system with an x-ray storage facility, as illustrated in Figure 4.8, many organizations choose to digitize existing x-ray films as shown in Figure 4.9 to avoid restrictions on clinical practice.

We intuitively feel that the longer-term advantages of teleradiology and digital storage of x-rays make greater sense and that an integrated electronic patient record will provide the networking platform to support distributing x-ray and other images to clinicians. Advances in technology, expansion of networks, and changes in clinical practice will make digital storage of x-rays happen. The question is, when? The decision analysis is a simple one that involves thinking of cost, practicality, and return on investment. The cost of trying to break this new ground when the technology is immature can quickly become colossal. We advise organizations to stay with the front-runners and be able to implement new advances quickly when they are tried and tested but not to be too adventurous and run the risk of breaking the bank in the process of trying to be the first.

Security Issues in Telehealth

The expensive and sought after high-tech equipment used by telehealth programs attracts theft. Hospitals and health care clinics are frequently difficult places to maintain security. Protecting telehealth systems from theft is an important operational consideration for telehealth programs. Simple housekeeping aspects of equipment security involve marking equipment so that it can be traced, keeping records of hardware identification numbers, physically restraining equipment to make it difficult to move, locking consulting rooms, installing antitheft devices, and getting adequate insurance coverage for equipment. These are all relatively simple considerations, and most well-managed health care organizations will already have operational policies to cover equipment security. Existing operational and insurance policies are usually readily adaptable to include telehealth equipment.

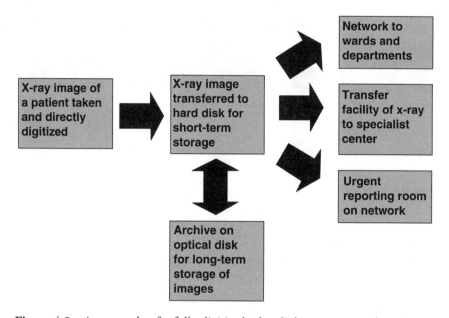

Figure 4.8 An example of a fully digitized teleradiology system with an image storage facility.

In addition to these hardware security concerns there are more complex data security considerations. Passwords are required to prevent unauthorized access to telehealth systems. As telehealth hardware becomes increasingly personal computer-based, these systems—and any access onto intranets and extranets through them—must be controlled. Among other things, these data security considerations include preventing unauthorized access to the system, stopping corruption of computer hard disks, constructing firewalls to secure networks, and blocking viruses from getting into the system. These security features of a telehealth service should all be manageable by linking the telehealth program with the network administration policies of the health care organizations with which they work. Unfortunately, when telehealth programs work alongside health care providers, they often find existing data security arrangements are far from ideal.

It is imperative to be obsessional about preserving data security in telehealth because of the risk management issues:

- Confidentiality of patient data must be maintained.
- The correct identity of health care professionals must be ensured.
- The legal and credentialing status of the health care professionals to practice in health care must be verified.

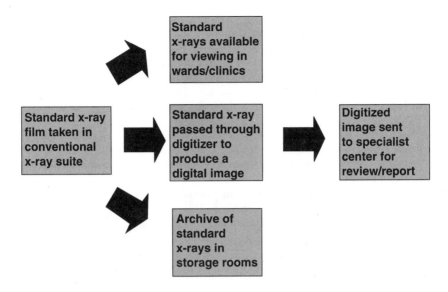

Figure 4.9   Partial digitization of x-ray images using a digitizer.

When telehealth projects are small and all the clinicians involved know each other, these risk management issues are usually neither recognized nor formally addressed. When telehealth programs expand and spread their geographical sphere of influence, they begin working with outside organizations. Clinical security quickly becomes a major risk management issue. Previous failure to adequately address clinical security considerations can often severely restrict the commercial prospects of telehealth programs when they try to expand service delivery. Having to go back and address these basic issues can deter potential investors and harm the prospects of an otherwise promising telehealth program. The clinical security issues often center on who at the remote site can initiate a telehealth transaction and who at the specialist center can receive and then conduct a telehealth transaction. Issues such as these translate into a series of questions that a telehealth program or company must ask. Viewed from the perspective of videoconsultation, these questions are shown in Table 4.6.

Laypeople have successfully impersonated doctors in conventional clinical settings. Telehealth programs must ensure that impersonation of doctors cannot take place, either intentionally or mistakenly. We know of instances where domestic cleaning staff who happened to be in a consulting suite initially answered a videoconsultation when no security precautions were in place. Unfortunately, some practitioners have committed fraud in billing for services and time using conventional methods of practice.

Table 4.6   Clinical Security Questions for Specialist
and Remote Centers in Teleconsultation

- Does the telehealth system restrict access to specialist consultation to users at centers with whom the telehealth program/company has a contractual arrangement?
- Does the telehealth system record data about any teleconsultations taking place that include a log of details about who teleconsults with whom, for how long, and for what reason?
- Does the telehealth system have passwords assigned that control which people are able to access the video conferencing system and undertake teleconsultations?
- Does the telehealth system allow open access to telecommunications network so that dial-up is possible to anywhere?
- Are clinical decisions made in teleconsultations clearly recorded, and are the remote site and specialist center contributions to these decisions clearly attributable?
- Are there mechanisms to ensure that clinicians at both the remote and specialist centers are correctly identified and appropriately licensed to practice?

Telehealth systems must have facilities for the monitoring and auditing of all teleconsultations. This is necessary for contracting, quality control, and risk management. Not to have these systems exposes a telehealth program to the possibility of fraud, for example, by allowing unauthorized consultation by clinicians for which they subsequently receive payment. Operational policies and procedures for the security and risk management of telehealth are essential when a telehealth program or company gets seriously into the business of delivering health care services. This means that any remote and specialist centers conducting telehealth transactions with one another must have service-level agreements as the basis for clinical contracting. These agreements must include specifying how each party in the teleconsultation ensures that clinicians are bona fide and appropriately licensed to practice.

Measurement of Clinical Quality
in Telehealth Transactions

Telehealth is potentially a high-risk area for clinical negligence and litigation claims against health care organizations adopting it. Allocation of clinical responsibility for patients between remote sites and the specialist center is often blurred. Consequently, there is a danger of telehealth consultations becoming a kind of clinical fishing expedition; if the remote site is unsure of the patient's diagnosis, unclear about the clinical findings, and unable to interpret the investigations, the specialist center is effectively being asked to take over the total management of the patient. In such situations it is often most appropriate to transfer the patient elsewhere to be managed and not to use telehealth. Telehealth transactions should have clear aims and objectives. The best way to achieve this is to use well-defined clinical protocols/guidelines in which the clinical management objectives are clearly outlined. Clinical protocols and guidelines that have set clear aims and objectives to their telehealth transactions usually include the following principles:

- The protocols and guidelines are based on establishing a working diagnosis derived from clinical findings.
- The protocols and guidelines offer physicians clear reasons for using telehealth, reasons based on clarifying the diagnosis, interpreting investigations, helping to decide a plan of management, reviewing the progress of treatment, and deciding when to transfer patients.
- They provide a clear understanding of the role and responsibilities of clinicians at the specialist center—in particular whether they are being asked to make a clinical decision about management, provide technical advice, give a second opinion, or offer scientific evidence to help frame clinical decisions for patients.
- Through the protocols and guidelines clinicians gain a clear understanding of what outcomes are expected from the telehealth transaction.
- Plans for any follow-up are specified, and under what circumstances.
- Guidelines and protocols make clear how the telehealth transaction is to be reimbursed.

Developing clinical protocols/guidelines in telehealth requires the active participation of clinicians at the remote sites and at the specialist center. This participation gives the protocols/guidelines organizational credibility and increases the likelihood that they will be used in routine practice. Clinical protocols/guidelines should include clinical standards included as quality measures in service-level agreements that specify exactly the telehealth services to be provided. Service-level agreements must outline when and how these quality standards should be audited. As well as working as external review mechanisms the protocols/guidelines can include a timetable for regular review of the quality of services by clinicians at both the remote sites and specialist centers. This review process must include explicit mechanisms for feedback of results to clinicians and managers so that services can be changed when necessary. Managers must be included in the quality review process so that contracts can be amended and the cost implications of any recommended changes to clinical practice can be readily identified.

Comfort, Convenience, and the Location of Telehealth Services for Patients

We have repeatedly stressed how important it is to have a customer/patient focus in telehealth. This patient focus not only applies to the clinical management of patients. It also applies to ensuring the comfort and convenience of patients who use telehealth services. Table 4.7 gives common areas of comfort and convenience for patients relevant to when they receive telehealth services. Although telehealth may streamline the process of delivering care in the eye of professionals and managers of health care systems, it does not always follow that services are improved for patients. A mother may find it more convenient to take a sick child to the emergency room and wait there to be seen instead of using a primary care facility with telehealth, which may involve booked appointments and delays in being seen and treated.

If investigations (e.g., ultrasound scans in pregnancy) are sent elsewhere for reporting, it can create delays. Patients may have to return for a follow-up visit to get a definitive report. If there are delays with telehealth, these must be justified by patient benefits, such as an improved quality of service or saving on travel time. When patients have to return later for results, it is often necessary to provide them with more than just a report. Depending on the clinical circumstance, education, counseling, and treatment may be required. This must be included in the service specification.

Problems with the sound cards on teleconsultation systems or the teleconsulting room acoustics can cause echoes, reverberation, and other sound distortions. These can make the teleconsultation unpleasant for patients and are often annoying and troublesome to correct. It is important that the problems are resolved because patients will vote with their feet and refuse a teleconsultation if they experience discomfort with poor sound quality. The etiquette of the teleconsultation must ensure that this takes place in comfort and privacy for patients. Easily adjustable chairs, comfortable examination couches, and lights that are not too bright are basic but necessary considerations. When a teleconsultation begins, patients must be informed of the identity of everybody present, including people at the remote site who can see the teleconsultation. Patients must give permission for anybody else to be present during the teleconsultation.

A convention in health care is that patients are clear about who is "their doctor" and "their nurse." When using telehealth, it must be equally clear to patients who is taking responsibility for all aspects of their care. Telehealth requires a therapeutic relationship between a patient and the practitioners involved in the teleconsultation. The relationship between the patient and the primary care physician or nurse practitioner at the remote site has to be

Table 4.7   Patient Convenience Considerations for Telehealth Services

* Do patients get their problems resolved faster by using telehealth?
* Is an investigation reported more quickly or is it of superior quality when using telehealth?
* Is the audio component of the teleconsultation of high enough quality?
* Does the teleconsultation take place in comfort and privacy?
* Are patients clear about where responsibility lies for all aspects of their care?
* Does telehealth allow patients to develop relationships to use in negotiating their choice about health care services?
* Do the aspects of a patient's health care that use telehealth interface well with other ways patients are receiving health care?
* Are there clear methods for patient feedback of suggestions and complaints about the telehealth program?

actively developed. In this relationship the practitioner should aim to act as a friend and counselor who does not expect to have the answers to all a patient's problems. Patients must understand that telehealth is a way for a clinician to contact other clinicians who may have the solutions. Telehealth services must deliver solutions that fit into the rest of the processes of care that patients need. For example, if a teleradiology program establishes a mammography service to screen women in remote rural areas for breast cancer, it is not sufficient just to perform the investigation and then report back on the mammogram. The telehealth program must also ensure women have access to counseling and biopsy if the results are abnormal.

Telehealth consultation facilities must be situated in convenient places for patients to use. In primary care settings this should be in a safe neighborhood where there is convenient transportation. If the teleconsultation center is in a hospital, it should be where patient access is easy. Space is often at a premium in hospitals, and telehealth programs are sometimes offered free space in inconvenient parts of a building. The most logical place to put the telehealth consultation suite in a hospital is often closely attached to the outpatient/ambulatory care department. As with other areas of health care delivery, telehealth programs must actively canvass patient views on the quality of services provided. Is the service comfortable, convenient, and acceptable to patients? If patients have complaints about their treatment, these responses must be acknowledged by the telehealth program and used as constructive feedback to further develop the service.

Backup and Fail-Safe Procedures

The main reasons for introducing a telehealth system into health care is that it provides a service that

- is deliverable at lower cost
- is of higher quality
- expands the market for health care delivery

Achieving these objectives when introducing a telehealth system usually means changing the existing ways of delivering health care. For example, if a telehealth service offers teleradiology and a teleconsultation facility to a remote trauma center, it may allow primary care physicians or nurse practitioners to staff this instead of trauma physicians and radiologists. In this situation the business case for telehealth results from the cost savings of deploying different grades of staff. If the new remote trauma center can deliver the service safely only if supported by telehealth, what happens if the telehealth link fails? The operational management of the telehealth service must include procedures to be instituted in case of a systems failure, such as those shown in Table 4.8. The roles and responsibilities of the emergency technical support for a telehealth system must be incorporated into clear policies in advance of a problem occurring. An in-house emergency technician may be required to establish where the problem lies, as illustrated in Table 4.9. Once a fault is located, there must be predefined maintenance agreements for emergency call-out and restoration of the service, agreements that are clearly established and accessible whenever required in an emergency situation.

Training of Practitioners

Practitioners have to be trained to conduct telehealth transactions. This training is needed to teach the practical aspects of using the equipment (cameras, etc.) as well as the clinical aspects of making remote diagnoses. A telehealth program must apportion a budget for the training and education of practitioners and adapt duty rotations to allow time to be taken for training. A useful training device for a telehealth program to consider is the temporary assignment of staff from the remote site to the specialist center and vice versa. Regular feedback to staff of information from clinical audit and outcomes measurement is an important element in the training of clinical staff to use telehealth effectively and efficiently.

Clinical training for staff at the remote site can take place from the specialist center using the telehealth system. This training can occur in an ad hoc manner, as and when required, or it can take place as part of the planned professional development of clinical staff. The training and education of staff should be seen as a vital part of any telehealth program and the appropriate policies developed. Many of the operational problems faced by telehealth services can be traced back to inadequate staff training. If telehealth is to

Table 4.8   Actions to Take If a Telehealth Service Fails

• Temporary cessation of the service and rerouting of patients
• Emergency transfer of patients where there is diagnostic doubt
• Back-up equipment
• Call-out of emergency technical support

augment routine health care delivery, organizations must have a strategy for how they train a competent telemedicine/telehealth workforce.

Educating Patients and Marketing a Telehealth Service

Patients as well as practitioners should be educated about telehealth and teleconsultation. Part of the operational management of telehealth services is therefore to market the service to the local population who will use the service. It is better that patients know about the telehealth service in advance, rather than learning about it when they need care and may feel anxious. Ways of marketing a telehealth service will depend on the particular type of service and its location. Many hospitals and health care providers are eager to market telehealth services because it shows that they are innovative and proactive organizations. Ways in which information about a telehealth service can be passed on to prospective patients of the service and marketed more widely are shown in Table 4.10.

THE FUTURE OF TELEHEALTH TRANSACTIONS

Health care services revolve around a vast number of processes, predominantly involving people. The professional training of doctors, nurses, physiotherapists, occupational therapists, physicians assistants, and others has been traditionally aimed at producing autonomous professionals. Groups of health care professionals usually work together within a single institution. The management challenge of introducing telehealth into existing health care settings is how to replace existing "people processes," involving health care professionals working in familiar ways, with a telehealth service that involves these professionals working in new ways. At the moment, the uptake and

Table 4.9   Problem Areas for Technical Failure of Telehealth Services

• The teleconsultation system at the remote site
• The local area network/wide area network
• The long-distance carrier's digital connection/network
• Another site's telehealth equipment

Table 4.10   Ways of Marketing Telehealth Services

* National and local television news reports
* National and local newspapers
* Posters and flyers put up locally
* Advertisements
* Information in newsletters
* Patient information materials
* Local meetings
* Direct word of mouth from other staff

use of telehealth is patchy, so the future of telehealth transactions is difficult to extrapolate from analyzing existing telehealth activity.

A real understanding of the future potential of telehealth transactions in health care comes from looking at how processes in health care currently requiring people will be enhanced and in some cases replaced by telehealth. We are at an early stage in the "process reengineering" of health care systems. The success of this change depends on introducing a critical mass of new information technology and networking capacity into health care, and this includes telehealth. Currently, the situation of telehealth is analogous to the telephone at the beginning of the 20th century. The telephone was a wonderful invention, but to be the only person with a telephone was of dubious benefit. The process of disseminating the telephone began from developing point-to-point connections. The real expansion of telephone use happened later when networks were established.

Telehealth is still at the stage of making point-to-point connections within individual organizations. At present a primary care doctor or a nurse practitioner wanting to initiate a teleconsultation with a dermatologist may have to do so by booking a future appointment slot and then bringing the patient back to teleconsult. This delay limits the immediacy of teleconsultation and therefore its benefits in routine clinical situations. As more centers offer telehealth services, they can begin to move away from point-to-point connections and network the services they can collectively provide. If seven medical centers all provide teledermatology services, then the logistics of providing a routine on-line dermatology consultation service can become a feasible proposition.

The population served by a health care organization is usually based on a defined geographical area. Some health care organizations also act as regional, supraregional, national, and international centers. These major centers depend on patients traveling to them to receive specialist care. Telehealth makes it possible for people to access health care from specialist centers without having to travel long distances and visit the center in person. In the future we can anticipate that the parents of a child with a rare form of leukemia in Cardiff, Wales, may be able to get advice on the management of this condition from the world expert in New York. The remote management of the child will include direct teleconsultation; telepathology to review the pathological results; telereradiology to check x-rays, CT, and MRI; and routine review of the hematology. Local care of the child, including the provision of drugs, routine investigations, information giving, and counseling can all take place close to home and be done by a local health care provider who works in collaboration with the specialist center in accordance with agreed on protocols/guidelines.

We are therefore likely to see that one effect of telehealth will be to fragment processes for delivering health care services as we currently recognize them. This fragmentation will in turn have a major effect on the institutions that deliver health care and the way in which the people inside these institutions will work in the future. The hospital is currently the single most important institution involved in bringing together the various processes for delivering health care services. Hospitals often expect to provide a portfolio of general medical services, including emergency care, general medicine, radiology, general surgery, orthopedics, pediatrics, oncology, obstetrics, dermatology, and otorhinolaryngology (ears, nose, and throat). Telehealth will allow the delivery of these services to be split from each other and therefore be less dependent on a single hospital as the primary source for their delivery.

This change of the hospital as an institution has parallels in areas of society outside medicine. The car factory used to produce all the component parts of the car, either in one factory site or brought in from local suppliers. This self-sufficiency of production meant that the car factory was relatively self-contained. In the past 20 years car factories have changed, becoming assembly centers where components produced in different parts of the world are put together to produce cars. In the early 1970s it seemed inconceivable that large car factories would change in that way. By the same token it is difficult to comprehend how large hospitals will change in the near future through a redefinition of the processes of care that telehealth promises.

If these changes are going to happen—that is, health care services will fragment and change from the way they are currently delivered—then the nature of telehealth transactions will also have to change. The methods of reimbursement for telehealth services must alter to provide the revenue sources on which the business cases to drive change must be based. The terms and conditions of employment for health care professionals must change to accommodate to the new ways in which health care will be delivered with telehealth. In the past, processes for delivering health care have been unclear and left to the individual discretion of autonomous health care professionals. Processes in health care will be codified and organized to provide telehealth efficiently.

The assembly of a car is now a complex logistical process involving just-in-time computer software to gather components from all over the world at the right time, in the right quantity and quality, and in the same place. In a similar way the delivery of health care in a more fragmented system will depend on critical processes bringing together the correct services, when and where these are required, processes that must be formalized in procedures and policies for the delivery of care. The real challenge for telehealth is not so much technological as technical. It is about the management of technical processes to marry information technology systems and clinical care into convenient, effective, high-quality methods for delivering health care efficiently and humanely to people who need it. The hallmark of a telehealth service that will deliver this future vision of telehealth transactions is having the policies and procedures in place to manage operational services effectively. The business of telehealth will involve delivering "just-in-time" health care services.

XML

Extensible markup language (XML) is a newly emerging authoring language (markup language) used in the creation of Web documents. XML and its ongoing development is a major area to watch in the evolution of telehealth. The importance of XML is that it helps to define data and facilitates its exchange free of the rigid constraints of the traditional to these activities of the database. Using an XML server it is possible to draw together data from disparate data sources from within the same or other organizations and then reformat these data onto XML and make them available for exchange. This is a way for organizations hampered by older legacy systems to move forward with information storage.

The importance of XML is that it "tags" data elements and makes these data more readily available to search engines. In effect, using XML creates unique identifiers that attach to data allowing data from previously incompatible information systems to be drawn together. As yet there are no agreed-upon standards for XML. Organizations such as American Health Standards Institute and Health Level Seven (HL7) are working to reach consensus. An initiative to promote XML started by Microsoft Corp is BizTalk. BizTalk establishes guidelines for the schemas that programmers use in tagging data elements. The development of agreed standards is crucial. Without them, similar data elements from two systems may have different tags. An analogy to the effect this could have was the crash of the Mars probe in 1999, which appeared to be due to the engineers involved in one part of the project using metric measurements and another group using imperial measures. The numbers were the same but what each denoted was radically different. Imagine the consequences of similar mismatches in clinical data applications involving hundreds of thousands of patients.

We are seeing a migration of health informatics onto the Web. Using HTML as the authoring language is time-consuming and laborious, XML promises to revolutionize this process. XML may be the crucial building block that enables the clinical patient record to interface with video-conferencing, the telephone consultation, and the facsimile to construct automated and transferable multimedia patient records, which we believe are the future basic building blocks of telehealth, and lend themselves to the true patient-based patient record—records that patients themselves can hold also.

POLICIES AND PROCEDURES FOR THE DELIVERY OF TELEHEALTH SERVICES

The delivery of health care services involves actively managing complex organizational tasks. The management of these tasks is increasingly based on formal policies and procedures that must be devised, communicated to patients and staff, and then revised to meet changing circumstances. Telehealth programs and companies must have explicit processes to manage the health care services they are delivering. Telehealth programs must therefore either devise their own policies and procedures or dovetail their services into policies and procedures already existing in the health care organizations with which they work. A list of common policies a telehealth provider must have is given in Table 4.11.

Table 4.11   Common Policies and Procedures Required in Telehealth

- Claims management and litigation
- Clinical audit
- Clinical care pathway development
- Clinical complaints
- Clinical risk management
- Contracting
- Drug and prescribing protocols
- Equipment procurement
- Infectious disease control
- Information network management (LAN, intranets, extranets)
- Marketing of services to patients and to staff
- Outcomes measurement
- Professional development
- Public relations
- Quality initiatives
- Research and development
- Service development
- Training and education

5

Telehealth Services

With an ever-increasing knowledge base about how telehealth works in routine health care delivery, it seems that many more clinical services can benefit from introducing telehealth into the care delivery process. Telehealth can help reengineer the way almost all areas of health care are configured in the future. When an organization considers the wide range of possible applications for telehealth, it should not be seduced by the technology into thinking telehealth's place in health care is self-evident. The current climate facing health systems in the United States, United Kingdom, New Zealand, Australia, and Canada means that telehealth applications must earn their right to a place in the care delivery process. For telehealth to earn this place it must offer positive advantages. As a minimum requirement it must either improve the quality of health care or increase access of people to health care services. This is still not enough. It must accomplish these goals at the same or at lower cost than conventional ways of delivering care and must not raise professional objections that make it impossible to implement. This formula for the success of a telehealth is shown in Figure 5.1

In this chapter we look at the current portfolio of telehealth applications from the critical perspective of what makes them successful and what factors may influence their ongoing development. These success criteria include the advantages to patients and clinicians of adopting teleconsultation instead of continuing with customary forms of consultation.

$$\textit{Telehealth Project's Success} = \frac{\textit{Quality of service and access to health care service}}{\textit{Cost of service and professional objection}}$$

Figure 5.1   A formula for success in telehealth.

TELEPATHOLOGY

Clinical Rationale for Providing Telepathology Services

Diagnostic pathology is a vital clinical support service to which any organization providing general or specialist hospital services usually must have ready access. Diagnostic pathology requirements cover a wide range of medical disciplines. The reports provided are from examinations of biological fluids, cell samples, and tissue specimens. An abnormal report can be due to a variety of pathological lesions, such as those listed in Table 5.1.

The diagnostic pathology report often can determine the diagnosis and subsequent treatment a patient requires. Making this diagnosis accurately, definitively, and as rapidly as possible is important to the patient, the clinician treating the patient, and the hospital. The pathological diagnosis may decide whether surgery is recommended to a patient and also what kind of surgery is needed, such as whether the optimal treatment for a woman with breast cancer would be to have her breast removed. Depending on a patient's condition and other clinical findings, samples of fluid, cells, or tissue for pathological analysis may require either routine or urgent examination. An accurate pathological result is critical to the patient's prognosis because it ensures that an accurate diagnosis is made and the appropriate treatment (surgery, radiotherapy, etc.) is then performed. Delay in making an accurate diagnosis may result in

- Delay in the patient's treatment that affects his/her chances of health/ survival
- A patient having two operations instead of one
- Avoidable distress to a patient and his/her relatives

Diagnostic pathology services are usually either general or specialized. Pathologists working in each type will have differing abilities to make a definitive pathological diagnosis depending on what kind of tissue is presented to them and what abnormality is present. Particular pathologists and particular diagnostic pathology departments develop their unique expertise from repeatedly seeing the same kinds of pathological abnormalities and yet

Table 5.1   Some Pathological Abnormalities

* Infective, e.g., syphilis
* Degenerative, e.g., Alzheimer's disease
* Traumatic, e.g., a hematoma
* Benign tumors, e.g., a lipoma
* Malignant tumors, e.g., breast cancer
* Metabolic problems, e.g., gout
* Congenital lesions, e.g., a dermoid cyst
* Chronic inflammatory, e.g., rheumatoid arthritis
* Acute inflammatory, e.g., acute appendicitis

being aware of all the other possible diagnoses. General hospitals usually employ general pathologists who are able to make a high proportion of pathological diagnoses themselves and refer any samples whose diagnosis they are unsure about to a specialist for a further opinion. In the conventional process of diagnostic triage, samples with diagnostic doubts have to be physically sent to one or more expert centers, where a definitive diagnosis is made, as shown in Figure 5.2.

The clinical rationale for telepathology as a means of cost-effectively replacing the physical transport of pathological specimens is that images of the slides can be transferred digitally instead of by transport systems (e.g., courier, airplane). The underlying presumption is that telepathology improves the quality of service offered to patients and increases their access to specialist services. In conventional pathological practice the time constraints associated with sending tissue specimens away for second opinions and waiting for a report can limit the use of outside second opinions.

The Business Case for Telepathology

There are usually three main areas in which a business case can be made to use telepathology; these are listed in Table 5.2. In the telepathology business case the scenario usually presented to a general hospital explains how it can replace part or all of its conventional diagnostic pathology services with telepathology services it buys from a remote provider. The business case for a general hospital considering whether to adopt telepathology has to be based on weighing the associated cost, quality, and organizational equation, as in Figure 5.1. This dictates that, to make it workable, the following must be considered:

* Quality and organizational factors and the cost of telepathology must be less than the cost of conventional pathology.

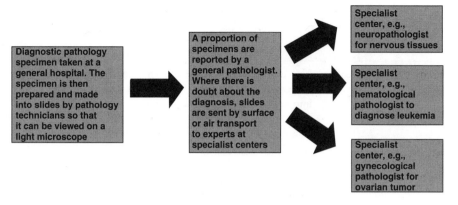

Figure 5.2   Conventional pathological diagnosis in a general hospital and obtaining second opinion, using physical transport.

- The quality of telepathology must be higher than that of conventional pathology services if cost and organizational factors are not considered.
- The organizational considerations are whether telepathology can replace a sufficient proportion of conventional pathology services to make it worthwhile adopting.
- Peer review of specimens on holiday cover are facilitated at remote sites.

These considerations are detailed in Tables 5.3, 5.4, and 5.5.

If a general hospital decides that it will use telepathology to bring in diagnostic expertise from pathologists at outside specialist centers to support its own general pathologists, it will inevitably add new capital and revenue costs to the expense of existing service. Making a business case for this can be difficult unless the use of telepathology to supplement the hospital's existing pathology service is viewed as a quality improvement measure that will indirectly reduce costs or increase business. Examples are (1) improving the efficiency of surgical services by better diagnosis and (2) attracting patient referrals by offering a unique service that competing local providers do not. When small hospitals consider contracting out all their diagnostic

Table 5.2   Usual Reasons to Support a Business Case for Telepathology

1. A general hospital restructures its conventional pathology department to enjoy economies from introducing telepathology.
2. A specialist center with diagnostic pathology expertise uses telepathology to market its services to a wider market.
3. A group of diagnostic pathologists form a physicians cooperative to market their expertise to clinics and general and specialist hospitals.

Table 5.3   Cost Factors in a Telepathology Case for a General Hospital

Factor in business case	A positive telepathology business case scenario	A negative telepathology business case scenario
Pathology service costs	The costs of the telepathology service take into account all the associated costs, not just the direct consultation costs. When these costs are analyzed, buying telepathology services from an outside provider is less expensive than providing these same services employing in-house staff.	The cost of buying telepathology services from an outside provider is higher than continuing to provide the service in house.
Telepathology equipment	The overhead cost of the repayments/depreciation of telepathology equipment is justified by the cost savings associated with the new service or by the additional revenue from new business generated by adopting telepathology.	The overhead cost of the repayments/depreciation of telepathology equipment cannot be justified because there are not sufficient savings or new business generated by adopting telepathology.
Telecoms line rental and call charges	The line rental and call charges of a telepathology service can be absorbed by the service and do not take the costs above the savings.	The line rental and call charges of a telepathology service take the costs above the savings.
General overhead costs	The overhead management costs, including billing, contract management, information technology, office space, and clerical support, can be absorbed by the service and do not take the costs above the savings.	The overhead and management costs take the costs of the telepathology service above the savings.

pathology consultation services to an outside telepathology provider, they should remember that they will still need to maintain a diagnostic pathology technical support facility to prepare slides and archive slides and reports for future reference and medicolegal protection.

Business cases for specialist centers aiming to provide telepathology services depend fundamentally on sufficient market interest among general

Table 5.4   Quality Factors in a Telepathology Case for a General Hospital

Factor in business case	A positive telepathology business case scenario	A negative telepathology business case scenario
Accuracy of pathological diagnosis	The diagnostic accuracy using telepathology must be high. If there are diagnostic doubts and further opinions are required, then processes must be in place for the transport and review of slides using conventional physical transfer systems. The rate of diagnostic mistakes must be equal to or less than conventional pathology services or it will harm patients and expose the service to the risks of lawsuits for clinical negligence.	The accuracy of diagnosis is not high enough to justify using telepathology instead of conventional pathology services based on direct light microscopical analysis by the pathologist.
Speed of pathological reporting	The time taken to get definitive reports for clinicians to use to initiate treatment and manage patients must be less than in using conventional pathology services.	Despite the speed of transfer of pathology slides the time taken to get a formal signed pathological report on which clinicians can act takes longer than conventional practice.
Access to diagnostic pathology	There is access to the required range of diagnostic pathology services to make telepathology a viable alternative.	There is not sufficient access to diagnostic pathology services to make telepathology viable because there has to be duplication of conventional services.

hospitals that they will be willing to refer cases and buy these services at the right price. The case for getting the diagnosis of carcinoma of the kidney or of a rare leukemia substantiated by a center with world authority, instead of by the local general hospital is an appealing proposition for patients. The current reality of the health care markets in the United States and the United Kingdom is that health insurers, HMOs, and health authorities make the actual decisions of what to purchase on behalf of patients. This situation makes purchasing diagnostic pathology advice from specialist centers by telepathology unlikely if its effect will be to increase the overall costs of providing health care. The two crucial issues for the specialist

**Table 5.5   Organizational Factors in a Telepathology Case
for a General Hospital**

Factor in business case	A positive telepathology business case scenario	A negative telepathology business case scenario
Importance of diagnostic pathology to the organization	Maintaining the current integrity of a diagnostic pathology department does not jeopardize another aspect of providing services, so the the process engineering to make the business case for telepathology can be successfully implemented.	Maintaining the current integrity of a diagnostic pathology department jeopardizes another aspect of providing services, e.g., the general pathologists may also provide a postmortem service. The hospital will still have to employ general pathologists irrespective of its need for histopathologists.
Clinical change management	The culture of the organization is amenable to change such as the introduction of a routine telepathology service.	The general culture of the organization will not accept the change telepathology will bring about, e.g., surgeons are not prepared to trust remote diagnosis and want the pathological expertise to remain in-house.
Backup and support for a telepathology service	There is a robust contracting system that can support a telepathology service and generate the revenue necessary to maintain the service. Associated clinical services such as clinical risk management, clinical audit, and coverage of clinical indemnity are available.	The contracting system is not robust enough to support the telepathology service. It is not clear how the income to sustain the service can be generated. Associated clinical services such as clinical risk management, clinical audit, and coverage of clinical indemnity are not there to cover the telepathology service.
Information technology backup and support	The organization has the capacity in house or from a facilities management service to provide the necessary information technology support for a routine telepathology service. The information technology backup is adequate to provide support in case of a systems failure, so services are clinically	The organization does not have the capacity in house or cannot buy at a reasonable cost from a facilities management service the expertise to provide the necessary information technology support for a routine telepathology service. The information technology backup is inadequate in case of a systems failure. The proposed service will be

Table 5.5   (Continued)

Factor in business case	A positive telepathology business case scenario	A negative telepathology business case scenario
Information technology backup and support *(cont.)*	safe and can fulfill contractual requirements.	unsafe clinically and cannot fulfill contractual requirements.
	The telepathology reporting system can interface with the normal mechanisms for clinical reporting and record keeping.	Providing a remote telepathology service is not compatible with efficiently interfacing with the normal mechanisms for clinical reporting and record keeping.

center wanting to market its diagnostic pathology services are the cost and the quality of the service they have to offer. Ultimately, the cost and quality of their service depends on how their clinical services are organized and the level of spare diagnostic pathology capacity they have available. Tables 5.6, 5.7, and 5.8 show the cost, quality, and organizational considerations a specialist center must consider in deciding whether it is feasible to establish a telepathology referral service.

A group of diagnostic pathologists who form a physicians' cooperative and market their expertise to general and specialist hospitals have essentially the same considerations in their business case as the one for the specialist hospital. The model for the way the pathologists can work together is that of a firm of lawyers in the United States or barristers in legal chambers in the United Kingdom. The main problem for the pathologists is to ensure that they have adequate management and billing processes in place and that they can access the necessary financial support. Delay in reimbursement can mean considerable delayed payment costs can accrue. For all three situations—the general hospital, the specialist center, and the physicians' cooperative—the initial question is whether there is evidence to support setting up telepathology services.

THE EVIDENCE FOR ESTABLISHING TELEPATHOLOGY SERVICES

Quality of Diagnosis

The primary factor in being able to offer a telepathology service is whether the diagnostic accuracy is high enough to make it clinically reliable. The two competing technologies for telepathology are static image and dynamic

**Table 5.6   Cost Factors for a Specialist Center
Offering Telepathology Services**

Factor in business case	A positive telepathology business case scenario	A negative telepathology business case scenario
Pathology service costs	The price charged to outside organizations for diagnostic pathology consultations must be competitive in the market and less than the price of getting diagnostic pathology services from conventional routes. Long-term, the costs of the service must be covered by the prices charged.	The specialist center can only offer a service at higher price than the costs of a conventional service to outside organizations, or there are other specialist centers that can offer the service at a lower price.
Telepathology equipment	The overhead cost of the repayments/depreciation of telepathology equipment are justified by the revenue generated from the new telepathology service.	When the overhead cost of the repayments/depreciation of telepathology equipment are added to the staff costs of the diagnostic pathologists, the price for the service is noncompetitive.
Telecoms line rental and call charges	The line rental and call charges of a telepathology service can be absorbed by the service and do not make the price to be charged noncompetitive.	The line rental and call charges of a telepathology service take the price to be charged above what is competitive in the marketplace.
General overhead costs	The overhead management costs, including billing, contract management, information technology, office space, and clerical support, can be absorbed by the service and do not take the price above what is competitive in the market.	The overhead and management costs take the price the telepathology service has to charge above what is competitive in the marketplace.

(real-time) image. In static telepathology the data from the pathological slides is sent from the remote site for storage at reading site and for later review. In dynamic telepathology the pathological image is viewed in real time, using video. In a study of static image telepathology involving 171 cases the diagnosis was correctly made in 74% of the cases.[113] The reasons for errors were inappropriate field selection, sampling biases of referring

**Table 5.7   Quality Factors for a Specialist Center
Offering Telepathology Services**

Factor in business case	A positive telepathology business case scenario	A negative telepathology business case scenario
Accuracy of pathological diagnosis	The diagnostic accuracy using telepathology must be sufficiently high to avoid doubts that require further opinion using conventional physical transfer of pathology slides. The rate of diagnostic mistakes must be equal to or less than conventional pathology services, or it will harm patients and expose the service to the risks of lawsuits for clinical negligence.	The accuracy of diagnosis is not high enough to justify using telepathology instead of conventional pathology services based on light microscopy.
Speed of pathological reporting	The time taken to get a definitive report that clinicians can use to initiate treatment must be less than in using conventional pathology services.	Despite the speed of transfer of images from pathology slides, the time taken to get a formal signed pathological report on which clinicians can act takes as long or longer than in conventional practice.
Access to diagnostic pathology	There is access to the required diagnostic pathology expertise to provide a dependable service that covers nights, holidays, and weekends if needed.	There is not sufficient expertise to cover the outside service, and the cost of hiring extra staff, if available, takes the price of the service above what the market will pay.

pathologists, and the tendency of static-image telepathologists to underestimate the complexity of cases. In a study of 52 neurosurgical frozen-section cases in which the referring pathologist selected appropriate fields for transmission to the consultant, 7 cases showed substantial disagreements.[114] A study comparing static image with dynamic image showed an overall diagnostic accuracy that was comparable (88% static vs. 90.5% dynamic).[115] In a study to investigate the accuracy of videomicroscopy of frozen sections, two pathologists reexamined 80 cases of archival material on which frozen sections had previously been performed; the examination showed that there were diagnostic errors. One pathologist made two false-negative diagnoses,

**Table 5.8   Organizational Factors for a Specialist Center
Offering Telepathology Services**

Factor in business case	A positive telepathology business case scenario	A negative telepathology business case scenario
Importance of diagnostic pathology to the organization	The future market projections for diagnostic pathology services favor the organization's investing in diagnostic pathology, this fits with the strategic direction of the organization.	The future market projections for diagnostic pathology services do not favor the organization's investing in diagnostic pathology. Or this investment does not fit with the strategic direction of the organization.
Clinical change management	Diagnostic pathologists are prepared to change their work practice to spend time in telepathology consultations instead of conventional light microscopy reporting. They are prepared to look at images on slides that have been prepared by outside organizations.	Diagnostic pathologists are not prepared to change their work practice sufficiently to make a telepathology service viable.
Backup and support for a telepathology service	There is a robust contracting system that can support a telepathology service and capture the revenues necessary to maintain the service. Associated clinical services such as clinical risk management, clinical audit, and coverage of clinical indemnity are available.	The contracting system is not robust enough to support the telepathology. It is not clear how the income necessary to sustain the service can be generated. Associated clinical services such as clinical risk management, clinical audit, and coverage of clinical indemnity are not available to cover the telepathology service.
Information technology backup and support	The organization has the capacity in house or from a facilities management service to provide the necessary information technology support for a routine telepathology service. The information technology backup is adequate to support in case of a systems failure so that services are clinically safe and can fulfill contractual requirements.	The organization does not have the capacity in house or cannot buy at a reasonable cost from a facilities management service the expertise to provide the necessary information technology support to offer a robust telepathology service. The information technology backup is inadequate to support in case of a systems failure. The service will be unsafe clinically and cannot fulfill contractual requirements.

Table 5.8   (Continued)

Factor in business case	A positive telepathology business case scenario	A negative telepathology business case scenario
Information technology backup and support (cont.)	The telepathology reporting system can interface with the normal mechanisms for clinical reporting and record keeping in outside organizations.	The telepathology service cannot efficiently provide clinical reports to outside organizations.

but no false-positive diagnosis. The other pathologist made one false-positive but no false-negative diagnosis. Using direct light microscopy, there had been no false-positive or false-negative diagnoses.[116]

The purpose of giving these data is to show that there can be appreciable diagnostic errors associated with using telepathology. Organizations considering offering commercial telepathology services must know their diagnostic accuracy rate. They must monitor that rate through meticulous clinical audit and offer only services in which they have demonstrable expertise. When organizations such as general hospitals plan to purchase telepathology services, they must know the diagnostic accuracy rate of any center they consider purchasing from and factor this into their decision. They should be cautious about accepting any figures quoted from the scientific literature as a proxy figure for actual data from the center from which they are considering purchasing. Both purchasers and providers of telepathology services should set contractual quality standards with rigorous and explicit quality control measures for their monitoring.

The Cost of Telepathology vs. Conventional Direct Light Microscopy

We are not aware of published data on the cost-effectiveness of telepathology. The way telepathology is currently practiced can vary widely from center to center. These variations all affect the costs of providing an operational telepathology service. The choice of whether a static or dynamic system is used in telepathology determines more than just the associated capital costs of equipment. It also affects the data transmission and the labor costs. This is because a major cost component of a telepathology service relates to the number of slides necessary to send to make a confident diagnosis. The data transmission requirements of the service relate directly to the number of slides that have to be sent. When making a conventional diagnosis using direct light microscopy, the pathologist first views the slide of a pathological specimen under low resolution and then selectively uses the higher-power objective to fully confirm the diagnosis. This low/high resolution examination with a static telepathology system may require the transfer of immense amounts of data to make a diagnosis.[117]

A dynamic telepathology referral requires less data transmission because the pathologist can first look at the slide under low resolution and then selectively choose the area where a higher resolution view is required. Consultants' examination times are significantly greater ($p < 0.001$) for this video microscopy.[118] Remote videomicrosopy examinations can be rapid consultations from the standpoint of the consultant, who may need to spend 2 minutes less per case to make the diagnosis. However, the referring pathologist/technician may have to spend 16 minutes per case selecting an average of 4.5 images for transmission to the consultant. To work in routine clinical practice, the use of remote videomicroscopy for pathology consultation means making a complex series of trade-offs involving cost, information loss, and timeliness of consultation.[114] These trade-offs can become complex if a telepathology service is to be economically feasible. Legal liability issues can become especially important if there is a high diagnostic error rate for telepathology. In some countries the diagnostic pathologist reading the slides is responsible for any errors introduced into the process by a remote technician, even when the technician is not the directly responsibility of or supervised by the consultant.[119]

TELEDERMATOLOGY CLINICAL RATIONALE FOR PROVIDING TELEDERMATOLOGY SERVICES

Dermatology is predominantly an office-based specialty and forms a major component of consultations in primary care. Shortages of dermatologists in the United Kingdom, the United States, and Canada mean that general practitioners, family physicians, and internists, rather than dermatologists, often see patients with skin diseases. The diagnostic accuracy for nondermatologists when they examine patients with skin diseases is only 54%.[120] Other evidence suggests that, even when skin lesions are correctly diagnosed, the patients are managed more appropriately and effectively by dermatologists.[121]

A presumption from this is that the treatment of people with skin diseases could be appreciably improved by giving them ready access to a dermatologist. The cost and logistics of making dermatology widely available are often prohibitive with conventional models of clinical practice. Consequently, hospitals in the United Kingdom have long waiting lists of people who want to see a dermatologist. In the United States, patients are often excluded from health care, including seeing a dermatologist, by lack of adequate health care insurance coverage. The incidence of skin disease, especially malignant melanoma, is rising, and therefore so is the demand for specialist dermatological advice. As a result, the need for skin biopsy is also growing.

As with telepathology, the important questions to consider in a business case for teledermatology services involve the cost, quality, and organizational ramifications of any change to services. Implementing any teledermatology service first depends on getting agreement to use teledermatology in place of an existing diagnostic and treatment service for patients with skin diseases, existing services usually provided either by primary care doctors or by a visiting dermatologist. Figure 5.3 shows how the conventional dermatology consultation fits into a more complex process for the delivery of care. Tables 5.9 to 5.14 show important factors to be considered in weighing the business case for teledermatology.

THE EVIDENCE FOR ESTABLISHING TELEDERMATOLOGY SERVICES

Quality of Diagnosis

Dermatology is a very visual medical specialty. Professional examinations such as the American Academy of Dermatology's specialty certifying exam and the membership of the Royal College of Physicians' exam in England use color slides to examine candidates. The basic principle of making a clinical diagnosis from photographs is therefore already instilled into dermatologists on both sides of the Atlantic.

There are two basic ways in which images are acquired for teledermatology—store-and-forward or real-time interactive videoconsultation. A difference exists between the quality of photographs of skin lesions taken by professional photographers and photographs taken by nonexperts in routine clinical practice. A difference in the quality of store-and-forward images was illustrated by a study in which nondermatologists and nonphotographers took the images transmitted for remote diagnosis: 27% were found to be unsatisfactory.[122] This same study showed that when office consultations resulted in certain diagnoses and high-quality photographs were sent, the remote clinicians agreed with the diagnosis in 75% of cases. Under less than ideal circumstances they concurred on their diagnoses only in somewhere between 61% and 64% of cases.

When 104 new patients with 135 dermatological conditions were referred to a dermatology clinic and examined with a videoconferencing system and

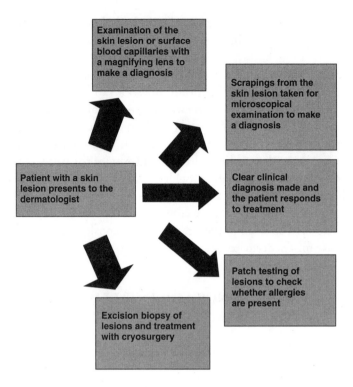

Figure 5.3   The extent of the dermatological consultation.

then by standard face-to-face consultation, 75% were correctly diagnosed by teledermatology. In the remainder a differential diagnosis was made in 7%, which agreed with the final diagnosis made later in a face-to-face consultation. In 12% the diagnosis was incorrect using the telemedicine system, and in 3% no diagnosis was made. Four percent of diagnoses could be made only when the patient was seen face to face.[123]

The Time Taken to Make a Diagnosis

The average time allotted for consultations in conventional dermatology outpatient visits differs, depending on the individual practitioner and the institution. On average, new patient appointments vary between 20 and 40 minutes, and follow-up visits last between 7 and 12 minutes. Teledermatology, using videoconsultation between a general practitioner and a dermatologist, took 5 to 10 minutes in 42% of cases, 15 minutes in 44% of cases, and more than 20 minutes in 14% of cases.[124]

Table 5.9   Cost Factors to Consider in Buying Teledermatology Services

Factor in business case	A positive teledermatology business case scenario	A negative teledermatology business case scenario
Dermatology service costs	The price for teledermatology services must be less than employing a dermatologist within the organization. If the price is no less or more, then the reduction in clinical risk, lower diagnosis/treatment costs, and/or any new business generated must justify the additional expense for the service. Long-term, the costs of the service must be fully covered by the prices charged.	Teledermatology services are more expensive than offering face-to-face consultations with a dermatologist. There is no rationale from reduced clinical risk, lower treatment/diagnosis costs, or generating new business to justify establishing a teledermatology service.
Teledermatology equipment	The overhead cost of the repayments/depreciation of teledermatology equipment are justified by the revenue generated, or costs saved by the new teledermatology service.	When the overhead cost of the repayments/depreciation of teledermatology equipment are added to the staff costs associated with dermatology consultancy the price for the service is not competitive.
Telecoms line rental and call charges	The line rental and call charges of a teledermatology service can be absorbed by the service without making the price that has to be charged uncompetitive.	The line rental and call charges of a teledermatology service take the price to be charged above what is competitive in the marketplace.
General overhead costs	The overhead management costs, including billing, contract management, information technology, office space, and clerical support can be absorbed by the service and do not take the price above what is competitive in the market.	The overhead and management costs take the price the teledermatology service has to charge above what is competitive in the marketplace.

Table 5.10   Quality Factors in a Teledermatology Case
for a General Hospital

Factor in business case	A positive teledermatology business case scenario	A negative teledermatology business case scenario
Accuracy of dermatological diagnosis	The diagnostic accuracy using teledermatology must be sufficient to avoid diagnostic doubts. This is particularly important in high-risk areas such as the diagnosis of malignant melanoma.	The accuracy of diagnosis is not high enough to justify using teledermatology instead of conventional methods of practice that may or may not include access to a dermatologist for face-to-face consultations.
	If there are diagnostic doubts about using teledermatology, they must be managed by introducing the appropriate clinical protocols and guidelines to ensure that patients with lesions that are not appropriate to manage with teledermatology are instead managed using conventional methods of treatment.	The necessary clinical guidelines and protocols cannot be devised or agreed to in order to implement a teledermatology program.
	The overall rate of diagnostic mistakes must be equal to or less than in dermatology taking place with conventional face-to-face consultations or it will harm patients and expose the service to the risks of lawsuits for clinical negligence.	
Speed of consultation	There must be an appointment booking system that allows patients to teleconsult in a convenient location and offer a teledermatology appointment within an acceptable time frame.	The logistics of establishing appointment schedules that allow patients to teleconsult at convenient times and places are not possible to arrange.
Access to teledermatology	There is access to the required range of diagnostic services, including microscopy, biopsy, and pathology.	There is not adequate access to the necessary diagnostic and treatment services that are required to make the teledermatology service a viable concern.

**Table 5.11   Organizational Factors in a Teledermatology Case
for a General Hospital**

Factor in business case	A positive teledermatology business case scenario	A negative teledermatology business case scenario
Importance of dermatology services	Switching the configuration of clinical services to provide teledermatology works as part of a portfolio of telehealth services the organization is developing. Dermatology is a weak area in the services that the organization is providing. Teledermatology offers a cost-effective way of enhancing the quality of services provided by the organization.	The current system for delivering dermatology services is well regarded by patients and clinicians and there is no product champion for introducing teledermatology.
Clinical change management	Clinicians in the organization are entrepreneurial and accepting of change and see teledermatology as a positive step for the organization. They support its development by referring patients they might otherwise have managed themselves.	The general culture of the organization will not accept changes such as teledermatology. Any gains from a teledermatology service, even if successful, are outweighed by the internal political difficulties this will induce in the organization.
Backup and support for a teledermatology service	The organization already has a robust contracting system that can support a teledermatology service and generate the revenue necessary to maintain the service. Associated clinical services such as clinical risk management, clinical audit, and coverage of clinical indemnity are available.	The contracting, marketing, and development systems cannot develop and sustain the income necessary for the service to survive. The organization does not have the capacity to cover clinical risk management, clinical audit, and clinical indemnity required by the teledermatology service.
Information technology backup and support	The organization has the capacity in house or from a facilities management service to provide the necessary information technology support for a routine teledermatology service.	The organization does not have the capacity in house or cannot buy at a reasonable cost from a facilities management service the expertise to provide the necessary information technology support for a routine teledermatology service.

Table 5.11   Organizational Factors in a Teledermatology Case for a General Hospital (Continued)

Factor in business case	A positive teledermatology business case scenario	A negative teledermatology business case scenario
Information technology backup and support (cont.)	The information technology backup is adequate to support in case of a systems failure so that services are clinically safe and can fulfill contractual requirements.	The information technology backup is inadequate to support in case of a systems failure. The service will be unsafe clinically and cannot fulfill contractual requirements.
	The teledermatology consultation system interfaces with mechanisms for microscopy and biopsy of specimens and also with clinical reporting and record keeping.	A remote teledermatology service cannot interface with other clinical processes efficiently and in ways that are convenient to patients.

The Cost-Effectiveness of Teledermatology

A comparison of dermatological treatment costs, using teledermatology instead of treatment by a primary care physician for 87 patients, showed cost savings associated with the teledermatology consultation.[120] In this study the average cost of caring for a diagnosed dermatological condition for all patients during an average period of 8 months prior to teledermatology diagnosis was $294, compared with $141 for the 6 months after diagnosis by teledermatology.

IS THERE A BUSINESS CASE FOR TELEDERMATOLOGY?

The vast majority of teledermatology programs in the United Kingdom, the United States, and Canada are grant-funded. As yet no definitive evidence exists to show a clear business case for teledermatology. Important issues to consider in making a teledermatology program into a self-sustaining, revenue-generating enterprise are given in Table 5.15.

In our opinion many current teledermatology programs are not yet seriously in the business of delivering health care. Duplication of effort by clinicians exists at both ends of the consultation, and the process of care is not streamlined to take advantage of the benefits of using telehealth.

Table 5.12   Cost Factors to Consider in Offering Specialist Teledermatology Consulting Services

Factor in business case	A positive teledermatology business case scenario	A negative teledermatology business case scenario
Dermatology service costs	The price charged for teledermatology services must be lower than the costs for other organizations of employing a full- or part-time, dermatologist in-house. If the price is no less or more, then the reduction in clinical risk, lower diagnosis/treatment costs, and/or any new business generated must justify the additional expenses of purchasing the services of the remote provider. The price must be equal to or less than competitive providers of the same quality. Long-term, the costs of the service must be fully covered by the prices charged.	The remote organization can provide services themselves in house or buy services from another provider more cheaply. There is no rational from reduced clinical risk, lower treatment/ diagnosis costs, or generating new business to justify establishing a teledermatology service. Or there are other specialist centers that can offer the service at a lower price.
Teledermatology equipment	The overhead cost of the repayments/depreciation of teledermatology equipment are justified by the revenue generated, from the sale of teledermatology consultations.	When the overhead cost of the repayments/depreciation of teledermatology equipment are added to the staff costs associated with offering dermatology consultancy, the price for the service is not competitive.
Telecoms line rental and call charges	The line rental and call charges of a teledermatology service can be absorbed by the service without making the price that has to be charged uncompetitive.	The line rental and call charges of a teledermatology service take the price to be charged above what is competitive in the marketplace.
General overhead costs	The overhead management costs, including billing, contract management, information technology, office space, and clerical support can be absorbed by the service and do not take price above what is competitive in the market.	The overhead and management costs take the price the teledermatology consulting service has to charge above what is competitive in the marketplace.

Table 5.13   Quality Factors in Offering Specialist Teledermatology Consulting Services

Factor in business case	A positive teledermatology business case scenario	A negative teledermatology business case scenario
Accuracy of dermatological diagnosis	The diagnostic accuracy of the teledermatology consultancy supplied must be of high caliber. There should be clear guidelines and protocols for the teledermatology consultancy advice supplied. These protocols must include the clinical conditions where it is appropriate for teledermatology to be used. If there are diagnostic doubts about using teledermatology, the guidelines must ensure access of patients to conventional methods of treatment. The error rate for teledermatology diagnosis must be audited and either equal to or less than conventional face-to-face dermatology consultations; otherwise it will harm patients and expose the service to the risks of lawsuits for clinical negligence.	The accuracy of diagnosis is not high enough to justify using teledermatology instead of conventional methods of practice. Any initial savings in costs are lost because of clinical indemnity claims or in having to include backup clinical systems. The necessary clinical guidelines and protocols cannot be devised or agreed to in order to implement a teledermatology program.
The speed of consultation	There must be an appointment booking system that allows patients to teleconsult in a convenient location and offers a teledermatology appointment within an acceptable time frame.	The logistics of establishing appointment schedules that allow patients to teleconsult at convenient times and places are not possible to arrange.
Access to teledermatology	There is access to the required range of diagnostic services, including microscopy, biopsy, and pathology.	The organization does not have adequate access to the necessary diagnostic and treatment services that are required to make the teledermatology service a viable concern.

Table 5.14   Organizational Factors to Consider for a Specialist Center Selling Teledermatology Services

Factor in business case	A positive teledermatology business case scenario	A negative teledermatology business case scenario
Importance of dermatology services	Switching the configuration of clinical services to provide teledermatology works as part of a portfolio of telehealth services the organization is developing. Dermatology is a weak area in the services that the organization is providing. Teledermatology offers a cost-effective way of enhancing the quality of services provided by the organization.	The current system for delivering dermatology services is well regarded by patients and clinicians, and there is no product champion for introducing teledermatology.
Clinical change management	Clinicians in the organization are entrepreneurial and accepting of change and will see teledermatology as a positive step for the organization and support its development by seeing patients remotely instead of in face-to-face consultations.	The general culture of the organization will not accept changes such as teledermatology. Any gains from a teledermatology service, even if successful, are outweighed by the internal political difficulties this will induce in the organization.
Backup and support for a teledermatology service	The organization already has a robust contracting system that can support a teledermatology service and generate the revenue necessary to maintain the service. Associated clinical services such as clinical risk management, clinical audit, and coverage of clinical indemnity are available.	The contracting, marketing, and development systems cannot develop and sustain the income necessary for the service to survive. The organization does not have the capacity to cover clinical risk management, clinical audit, and clinical indemnity required by the teledermatology service.
Information technology backup and support	The organization has the capacity in house or from a facilities management service to provide the necessary information technology support for a routine teledermatology service.	The organization does not have the capacity in house or cannot buy at a reasonable cost from a facilities management service the expertise to provide the necessary information technology support for a routine teledermatology service.

Table 5.14   Organizational Factors to Consider for a Specialist Center Selling Teledermatology Services *(Continued)*

Factor in business case	A positive telepathology business case scenario	A negative telepathology business case scenario
Information technology backup and support *(cont.)*	The information technology backup is adequate to support in case of a systems failure so that services are clinically safe and can fulfill contractual requirements.	The information technology backup is inadequate to support in case of a systems failure. The service will be unsafe clinically and cannot fulfill contractual requirements.
	The teledermatology consultation system interfaces with mechanisms for ordering microscopy and biopsy of specimens and also with clinical reporting and record keeping.	A remote teledermatology service cannot interface with other clinical processes efficiently and in ways that are convenient to patients.

TELERADIOLOGY: CLINICAL RATIONALE

From current clinical standpoints, radiology is the ideal clinical service for telehealth. The majority of x-rays are standard investigations performed in a standardized manner. Usually they are then reported in an almost "production line" process. For the majority of x-ray investigations, the radiologist reporting the x-ray does not have to be present when the investigation is performed. Patient clinical information and the reason for conducting the investigation are usually written on request forms by the practitioners making the referrals. Many small hospitals and clinics have no specialized x-ray examinations taking place yet require the presence of an on-site radiologist solely to report standard imaging. These hospitals and clinics are ideal settings for establishing teleradiology services. Their routine x-ray investigations can be performed and sent to a specialist hospital center for formal reporting. Unlike diagnostic pathology, in which the case for using telepathology is mainly to send the unusual cases for remote reporting, in teleradiology it makes sense to send the high-volume routine investigations for routine reporting. High-volume, low-cost procedures such as these can generate high revenues and make a strong business case to support teleradiology.

Good clinical and business cases also exist for using teleradiology to review specialist radiological investigations in clinical areas such as neurosurgery. The decision to operate on an acutely ill or injured neurosurgical patient often depends on the results of CT and MRI scans that can be transmitted

Table 5.15   Considerations in Establishing
a Commercial Teledermatology Service

- Clinical care must be based on clearly defined protocols that indicate what conditions can be safely managed by teledermatology and what the treatment pathways to be followed are, particularly when there is diagnostic uncertainty.
- The roles, responsibilities, and competencies of the clinicians at both ends of the teleconsultation must be set out.
- The teledermatology service specification must be clearly defined, with set standards that are regularly audited.
- The price for the service must be based on clear understanding of what the real costs attributable to the teledermatology service are, and these must be seen in the context of outcome measures that include progression or cure of the disease and patient satisfaction.

---

from the site of the investigation to the clinician. This is particularly useful when it is an after-hours investigation. Teleradiology can theoretically contribute to cost-effectiveness in the delivery of clinical care in three ways, as shown in Table 5.16. Figures 5.4 and 5.5 show how teleradiology improves the efficiency of care.

This simply illustrates how teleradiology can bring about the process reengineering of x-ray services and shows where the potential business case lies. Not only does teleradiology cut down the number of stages in the overall process by 25%, it also speeds up the transfer time between processes. Multiplying these savings over the thousands of x-rays taken each day in a busy x-ray department suggests how real cost savings can quickly accrue. These savings must be assessed in conjunction with other financial considerations, such as the capital investment required and the expenses of streamlining the process of handling radiology data instead of x-ray films to fully make a business case. The types of organizations that may benefit from adopting teleradiology are shown in Table 5.17.

As with pathology and dermatology the case for adopting telehealth in radiology can be reviewed in terms of the cost, quality, and organizational considerations that are shown in Tables 5.18, 5.19, and 5.20. Tables 5.21, 5.22, and 5.23 show the issues to consider for a specialist center interested in selling teleradiology services.

THE EVIDENCE FOR ESTABLISHING
TELERADIOLOGY SERVICES
Quality of Diagnosis

The evidence for the quality of diagnosis for teleradiology is conflicting because there are no agreed-on test materials on which to make objective

Table 5.16   Ways Teleradiology Improves the Cost-Effectiveness of Care

1. Teleradiology can reduce the costs of providing radiology services because of skills-mix changes that enable the process reengineering of these services.
2. Teleradiology can speed up the process of care by reducing the time from the clinician's request for an x-ray examination to receipt of the report.
3. Teleradiology can save on materials costs by reducing the need for x-ray film, processing chemicals, and archiving x-ray films.

comparisons. A study of a teleradiology link based on standard personal computers, a flat-bed CCD scanner and a 64 kilobits/sec dial-up digital integrated services digital network (ISDN) telephone line on 254 x-ray films (174 uncompressed, 80 compressed) showed 96% of the uncompressed images and 98% of the compressed images were technically acceptable. The total diagnostic agreement between the acceptable transmitted images and the original films was 98%. Image quality was sufficient for diagnosis in CT and conventional chest and bone radiographs.[125]

A study of the diagnostic capacity of emergency room physicians and radiologists on x-rays taken from the radiology library showed a statistical difference in the ability of each group to make an accurate diagnosis of digitized images presented on a workstation.[126] A Norwegian comparison of conventional radiology with teleradiology concluded that there were no significant differences between the two.[127] This confirmed the findings of an earlier study involving 685 clinical radiological investigations.[128]

The Cost of Teleradiology

A Norwegian primary care study in a remote rural area showed that conventional radiology was cheaper than using teleradiology; although teleradiology could not be justified on strict monetary grounds, it could be in terms of access to care.[129] The use of teleradiology to triage 100 neurosurgical patients in Pennsylvania and help decide whether or not they should be transferred to a neurosurgical center saved $502,638.[130]

The Business Case for Teleradiology

In a review of the teleradiology literature, grant-funded programs have demonstrated that teleradiology is feasible and acceptable in clinical practice. What they have not demonstrated is the business case underpinning routine commercial teleradiology. We know of no conclusive cost-effectiveness teleradiology studies. In the studies that have looked at the costs involved the financial data has been crude and difficult to interpret critically.

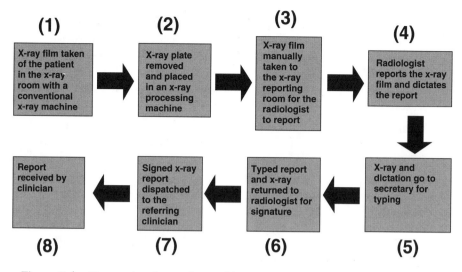

Figure 5.4   Conventional steps from taking an x-ray to receiving a report.

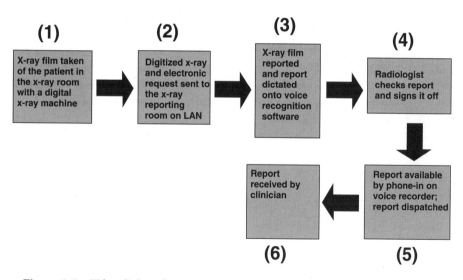

Figure 5.5   Teleradiology from x-ray to report.

The acceptability of teleradiology to the wide body of physicians has not yet been clearly demonstrated; neither has the business case for teleradiology been satisfactorily outlined. The expansion in commercial teleradiology would suggest that it is profitable. This raises an interesting paradox for the evaluation of telehealth in health care markets. If a teleradiology service develops a

Table 5.17   Typical Organizations that Benefit from Teleradiology

- Smaller hospitals or clinics that can either open a radiology department or streamline their existing service by sending x-rays elsewhere to be reported and therefore buying-in teleradiology services

- Large hospitals that have the staff and resources to run a remote x-ray reporting facility to service other organizations teleradiology needs

- Groups of radiologists that want to contract to hospitals a service for the reporting of x-rays

highly profitable model for service delivery, should it share this in the health services research literature for the greater good? Or should it capitalize on its ingenuity and go straight to developing a commercial service? Currently, it seems that teleradiology programs, like other areas of telehealth, must develop their own business case, based on a critical assessment of the diagnostic accuracy and quality of the actual teleradiology consultation service they provide and not on figures quoted from the scientific literature. The cost comparisons between teleradiology and conventional radiology must be calculated critically and should include all the costs attributable to the program.

TELEPSYCHIATRY

Telepsychiatry is a promising area of telehealth. It has been piloted with obsessive compulsive disorder,[131] child behavior disorders and family therapy,[132] and schizophrenia. Areas where telepsychiatry has been useful and effective are presented in Table 5.24.[133] As with teledermatology, the business case for telepsychiatry must be worked out from similar cost, quality, and organizational considerations.

TELESURGERY

Telesurgery is a glamorized area of telehealth often shown on television. There are currently four main areas where telesurgery is in common use:

- Telepresence surgery
- Telerobotics
- Telementoring
- Surgical training and education

Table 5.18   Cost Factors to Consider in Adopting Teleradiology

Factor in business case	A positive teleradiology business case scenario	A negative teleradiology business case scenario
Radiology service costs	The cost of digitizing x-rays to send away for remote consultation and buying the radiology consultations must be less than using conventional x-ray film and employing radiologists in house. Using teleradiology must lower clinical risk, lower diagnosis/ treatment costs, and/or generate new business to cover any additional expense for the service. Because radiology is a service specialty, the costs of the teleradiology service must be fully recovered within other contracts for clinical services. This may or may not require recharging other specialty users of radiology for the costs of the service.	A teleradiology service is more expensive than offering conventional radiology services with x-ray film and employing radiologists directly. There is no rationale from reduced clinical risk, lower treatment/diagnosis costs, or generating new business to justify establishing a teleradiology service. There is no internal customer process within the organization whereby the costs of the teleradiology service can be recharged to other specialty departments.
Teleradiology equipment	The overhead cost of the repayments/depreciation of teleradiology equipment are covered by the revenue generated or saved by the new radiology service.	When the overhead cost of the repayments/depreciation of teleradiology equipment are added to the remaining staff costs in the radiology department, the cost of running the service is too high to be sustainable.
Telecoms line rental and call charges	The line rental and call charges of a teleradiology service can be absorbed by the service without making the price that has to be charged for services uncompetitive.	The line rental and call charges of a teleradiology service take the price to be charged above what is competitive in the marketplace.
General overhead costs	The overhead management costs, including billing, contract management, information technology, office space, and clerical support can be absorbed by the service and do not take the price above what is competitive in the market.	The overhead and management costs take the price the teleradiology service has to charge above what is competitive in the marketplace.

Table 5.19   Quality Factors in a Teleradiology Case for a General Hospital

Factor in business case	A positive teleradiology business case scenario	A negative teleradiology business case scenario
Accuracy of radiological diagnosis	The diagnostic accuracy of teleradiology must equal conventional x-ray reporting. Although digitizing x-rays at the remote end can be cost-effective, reproducing x-rays at the reporting end as well has to be a business proposition. If there are consistent diagnostic doubts about teleradiology, these must be managed by developing appropriate clinical protocols and guidelines, ensuring that other investigations are used to confirm the diagnosis. Or patients must be triaged to ensure that investigations can be done elsewhere where there is less diagnostic doubt.	The accuracy of diagnosis is not high enough to justify using teleradiology instead of conventional methods of x-ray reporting. The necessary clinical guidelines and protocols cannot be devised or agreed to in order to implement a teleradiology program in which patients can be successfully managed. Backup systems for failed diagnosis are expensive in radiology. In some instances these can require sustaining processes that getting rid of formed the business case for the teleradiology program, e.g., maintaining an on-site radiologist's presence at the remote site.
The speed of consultation	There must be a teleradiology consultation request system ensuring that x-rays and requests are forwarded for reporting automatically. The reporting system must provide the signed report or its proxy as rapidly or more rapidly than conventional reporting systems.	The logistics of establishing automation of reporting does not speed up the ultimate delivery of reports to clinicians. Or the system is inconsistent and unreliable.
Access to teleradiology	Teleradiology improves the access of patients to x-ray services. Patients can get access to radiology services at local clinics and hospitals and avoid travel to large hospital centers.	The demand from the local population for local access to radiology services is not enough to justify teleradiology.

Table 5.20   Organizational Factors for Teleradiology in a General Hospital

Factor in business case	A positive teleradiology business case scenario	A negative teleradiology business case scenario
Importance of radiology services to the organization	There are no specific reasons why the organization needs to employ radiologists on site. Switching the configuration of clinical services to provide teleradiology is as efficient. Clinicians have a method of viewing x-rays throughout the organization, either on x-ray films or as digitized images on a LAN (local area network). If patients are transferred to other organizations there are ways to reproduce x-rays to send with the patient.	Teleradiology conflicts with the strategic direction of the organization. A need to provide specialist radiology, such as interventional radiology and radiology training scheme, mean that it is important that the organization retains its conventional radiology services.
Clinical change management	Clinicians accept the discipline of coming down to the radiology department or using computer terminals to view x-rays on the LAN instead of having plain x-ray films. Clinicians are prepared to work with radiologists at a remote site instead of having radiologists in house.	The general culture of the organization will not accept the changes imposed by introducing teleradiology. This means that the cost savings to support teleradiology will be difficult to realize.
Backup and support for a teleradiology service	The organization already has a robust contracting system that can support a teleradiology service and generate the revenue necessary to maintain the service. Associated clinical services such as clinical risk management, clinical audit, and coverage of clinical indemnity are available.	The contracting, marketing and development systems cannot develop and sustain the income necessary for the service to survive. The organization does not have the capacity to cover clinical risk management, clinical audit, and clinical indemnity required by the teleradiology service.

**Table 5.20   Organizational Factors for Teleradiology
in a General Hospital *(Continued)***

Factor in business case	A positive teleradiology business case scenario	A negative teleradiology business case scenario
Information technology backup and support	The organization already has a PACS (picture archive and communication systems) system or has the capacity in house or from a facilities management service to provide the necessary information technology support for a routine teleradiology service.	The organization cannot supply the IT (information technology) infrastructure to support a routine teleradiology service.

Telepresence Surgery

Telepresence surgery has its roots in the robotic arms used in the atomic energy industry to manipulate radioactive isotopes. This principle has been extended and linked to current computer technology. Surgeons are now able to operate on patients remotely using digital connections to a remote surgical interface. Force feedback (haptic) transmission to the surgeon uses servo-motors that give the sensation of "feel" to the remote surgeon.[134,135]

Telerobotics

Telerobotics[136,137] is essentially the same as telepresence except that the feedback from the servo systems is not included, so there is no haptic element to remote surgery. Telerobotics uses data transmission techniques to enable a remote surgeon to visualize and manipulate a remote surgical arm.

Telementoring

In telementoring[138] a surgeon at a primary operating site can consult another experienced surgeon or colleague if required during a surgical operation. This study used telementoring in complex laparoscopic cases, including upper pole nephrectomy, diagnostic laparoscopy with inguinal hernia repair, orchiectomy, gastric augmentation with bladder suspension, bladder reconstruction, and uretheral lithotomy. All the surgical procedures were accomplished successfully without intraoperative or postoperative complications.

Table 5.21   Cost Factors to Consider in Selling Teleradiology Services

Factor in business case	A positive teleradiology business case scenario	A negative teleradiology business case scenario
Radiology service pricing	The price charged to the remote center for teleradiology services is less than the cost for the remote site of employing a radiologist in house. If the price is more than this, then the reduction in clinical risk, lower diagnosis/treatment costs, and/or any new business generated justify the additional expenses charged for the service. Long-term, the costs of the service must be fully covered by the prices charged.	Teleradiology services are more expensive than the costs for remote organizations of continuing to provide the service. There is no rationale from reduced clinical risk, lower treatment/diagnosis costs or generating new business to justify establishing a teleradiology service. Or other organizations can provide teleradiology services more cheaply.
Teleradiology equipment	The overhead costs of the repayments/depreciation of teleradiology equipment are covered by the amount of revenue generated from the new teleradiology service.	The overhead cost of the repayments/depreciation of teleradiology equipment and staff costs of radiology consultancy make the price that has to be charged for the service uncompetitive in the market.
Telecoms line rental and call charges	The line rental and call charges of a teleradiology service can be absorbed by the service without making the price that has to be charged uncompetitive.	The line rental and call charges of a teleradiology service take the price to be charged above what is competitive in the marketplace.
General overhead costs	The overhead management costs, including billing, contract management, information technology, office space, and clerical support can be absorbed by the service and do not take price above what is competitive in the market.	The overhead and management costs take the price the teleradiology service has to charge above what is competitive in the marketplace.

Table 5.22   Quality Factors in Selling Teleradiology Services

Factor in business case	A positive teleradiology business case scenario	A negative teleradiology business case scenario
Accuracy of radiological diagnosis	The diagnostic accuracy of teleradiology services is as high or higher than conventional radiology. The accuracy of diagnosis is a selling point that helps justify the remote site buying the teleradiology service. The accuracy of diagnosis is monitored by regular audit and a quality assurance program that is fed back to organizations buying teleradiology services.	The accuracy of diagnosis will not be high enough to sell a robust teleradiology service to outside organizations.
Speed of consultation	There are well-organized processes in place for the reporting of x-rays from outside organizations. This process must include archiving x-rays and reports for medicolegal purposes as well as getting the reports back to the remote site as fast as or faster than conventional radiology car. The reporting system enables the remote site to query the teleradiology reports so that a remote clinician and specialist consultant can simultaneously view the x-ray image and discuss the diagnosis.	Although the teleradiology system may allow the transfer of x-ray data, it does not permit the efficient tracking, audit, and delivery of reports to the remote site.
Access to teleradiology	Dedicated T1 or ISDN lines give easy access for remote sites to the organization for teleradiology referrals. In the US there must be no state licensure problems to act as a barrier to the remote reading of x-rays.	There are problems for remote organizations to access the teleradiology service either because of data communication or licensure problems.

Table 5.23   Organizational Factors in Selling Teledermatology Services

Factor in business case	A positive teleradiology business case scenario	A negative teleradiology business case scenario
Importance of radiology services	Radiology is a major interest of the organization. The development of teleradiology fits with the future strategic direction for the organization. Switching the configuration of clinical services to provide teleradiology works as part of a portfolio of telehealth services the organization is developing. Radiology services are an important source of referrals from outside physicians to the organization. An efficient radiology service results in referrals to other specialties.	The current system for delivering radiology is established, and there is no product champion for introducing teleradiology. Other associated health care organizations are not interested in changing their services and purchasing teleradiology services.
Clinical change management	Clinicians in the organization are entrepreneurial and accepting of change. Radiologists are able to organize themselves so that reporting sessions for remote radiology can take place efficiently and they can cover the required sessions during the week and out of hours as required.	The general culture of the organization will not accept the changes to working practice that teleradiology demands. Any potential gains from a teleradiology service, even if successful, are outweighed by the internal political difficulties this will induce in the organization.
Backup and support for a teleradiology service	The organization has a robust contracting system that can support a teleradiology service and generate the revenue necessary to maintain the service. Associated clinical services such as clinical risk management, clinical audit, and coverage of clinical indemnity are available.	The contracting, marketing, and development systems cannot develop and sustain the income necessary for the service to survive. The organization does not have the capacity to cover clinical risk management, clinical audit, and clinical indemnity required by the teledermatology service.
Information technology backup and support	The organization has the capacity in house or from a facilities management service to provide	The organization does not have the capacity to provide the necessary

**Table 5.23   Organizational Factors in Selling
Teledermatology Services** *(Continued)*

Factor in business case	A positive teleradiology business case scenario	A negative teleradiology business case scenario
Information technology backup and support *(cont.)*	the necessary information technology support for a routine teleradiology service.	information technology support for a routine teleradiology service.
	The information technology backup is adequate to support in case of a systems failure so that services are clinically safe and can fulfill contractual requirements.	The information technology backup is inadequate to support in case of a systems failure. The service will be unsafe clinically and cannot fulfill contractual requirements.

Surgical Education and Training

Interactive videoconferencing programs are a way for surgical teams to receive the education and training to stay current in the rapidly changing world of operative surgery using the laparoscope.[139]

The Business Case for Telesurgery

Telesurgery usually represents the high cost, high technology end of the telehealth market. Examples of battlefield surgery, where soldiers are operated on in remote situations, are extremely impressive. What is less impressive in supporting the commercial future of telehealth is how much these can cost per case to perform. When we look around at successful high technology companies in the commercial and industrial sectors, their "recipe" for success often seems to be from developing high-volume, low-cost products. In

Table 5.24   Applications of Telepsychiatry[133]

- Initial evaluation, emergency care, and law enforcement referrals
- Preadmission and predischarge planning
- Medication management
- Follow-up care
- Evaluations and diagnostics
- Short-term case management
- Management of chronically ill patients
- Primary care physician consults
- Educational, administrative, and other clinical applications

Table 5.25   Promising Areas of Telehealth Development

- Telespirometry[140]
- Teleoncology[141]
- Neurology[142]
- Otorhinolaryngology[14]
- Teleophthalmology[143]
- Telemammography[144]
- Telehome care[145]
- Prison health care[18]
- Cardiology[146]

the near future we believe the success of telehealth will be based on the high-volume, low-cost telehealth applications. Telementoring is such an application in telesurgery.

OTHER CURRENT AREAS OF TELEHEALTH DEVELOPMENT

Table 5.25 outlines other promising areas of teleheath where it may be possible to make a business case for their introduction into routine clinical care. It is beyond the scope of this book to make a detailed case for introducing all these areas of telehealth. The principles outlined for telepathology, teledermatology, and teleradiology provide a framework to use with information about the markets and business of telehealth provided later to make this assessment.

6

Regulatory, Legislative, and Political Considerations in Telehealth

As well as the clinical and technical challenges of configuring a workable telehealth services there are regulatory, legislative, and political dimensions to consider. In this book we repeatedly emphasize the future potential of telehealth as a way of improving the standard of health care service delivery to the ordinary patients who are the ultimate consumers of health care. We have illustrated how telehealth offers possible solutions to what otherwise seem intractable problems for societies of how to maintain high quality health care for their populations at a time when the costs of health care continue to rise and heath coverage is falling. Unfortunately, these dynamics do not play out in the isolated world of health care; they affect other outside economic, professional, and political interests— interests that are all vying to influence the future for telehealth in market-driven health care systems in the United Kingdom, the United States, Canada, New Zealand, and Australia.

Telehealth often seems easy when an individual or an organization first thinks about using it to deliver health care services. Ideas are common. Taking an initial idea forward to the stage of a successful pilot project takes skill. The real prize is in taking an idea, or a pilot, to the stage of a robust and sustainable clinical service. This requires ingenuity.

After thinking through the operational details of clinical and technical delivery of services, a would-be telehealth provider organization has yet another layer of complexity to consider. This complexity includes legal, legislative and regulatory aspects that can ultimately decide whether a telehealth program has real commercial prospects. This complexity inevitably results because telehealth cuts across the traditional boundaries of many interest groups. These groups include

- Health care providers
- Professional organizations
- Telecommunications companies
- Government agencies
- Medical equipment suppliers
- Patient organizations
- Health insurers
- Clinical indemnity insurers

Groups like these often have interests of their own to consider, interests that may be programmed to either preserve or eliminate previous legislation. These groups may lobby to influence any proposed legislative changes in their favor. Introducing telehealth also confronts other entrenched positions including traditional professional barriers relating to the practice of health care. Dealing with these obstacles is rarely as simple as just reading the small print. Many of the legal, legislative, and regulatory issues in telehealth have yet to be fully worked through. Consequently there is often not even the small print for a telehealth program to consult. In this chapter we look at these legal, legislative and regulatory areas and assess their importance in defining strategies for future investment in telehealth. These are not areas where we can define a certain future. We predict that the survivors in telehealth who will emerge as major players in the future will be those who have a strong sense of these legal, legislative, and political agendas and use them to their advantage. It is worth pointing out that the "blue sky innovators" and "groundbreakers" in any field are often not the long-term survivors. A telehealth program's strategy for survival and growth must include the decision on whether to be at the leading edge, the trailing edge, or the bleeding edge.

LEGAL ASPECTS OF PROVIDING TELEHEALTH SERVICES

The precedents and specifics of much of the case law in relation to telehealth are in their infancy. The legal position of delivering health care remotely using telehealth has yet to be clearly established. Nonetheless, we believe all telehealth programs must always consider their legal position very carefully in advance. Some telehealth programs take a "wait and see" approach over legal issues, imagining telehealth is no different from conventional health care practice. We see this as a high-risk strategy, one that can put patients and the program at unnecessary risk. Some of the major legal issues we frequently find need consideration are shown in Table 6.1

How Is Clinical Responsibility Apportioned Between the Practitioner at the Remote Consulting Site and the Adviser at the Specialist Center?

If a patient is receiving care simultaneously from clinicians at both ends of a telehealth system, where does the clinical responsibility for the care of the patient lie? This question is of much more than academic interest to a health care organization using telehealth because of its implications in case of a medical malpractice suit. For example, if an obstetrician in the city provides remote obstetric advice to practitioner in a rural area and a child is subsequently brain-damaged from birth asphyxia, who is legally responsible? An obstetric claim for a six-figure sum against a telehealth provider could signal the end of the telehealth program unless it has adequate clinical indemnity cover. Obtaining this kind of clinical indemnity cover will now invariably require working out any clinical risk management issues carefully in advance.

An infinite number of combinations of possible clinical circumstances and of individuals can be involved in delivering remote health care. This makes a definitive ruling on the precise legal accountability of clinicians teleconsulting at the remote and receiving ends of a telehealth system unlikely to happen in the near future. Inevitably, we see each of the clinicians as having some degree of joint responsibility for the care of the patient. This sharing of responsibility would probably be reflected in any lawsuit. A lawsuit would likely be directed at both the clinicians and the organizations for which they work. The larger the financial resources of the organization, the more likely it will be included in a suit. In this current situation the best defense against a medical negligence claim associated with telehealth is to prevent it from happening. We discourage the use of telehealth as some kind of clinical fishing trip that encourages clinicians who are unsure of what is happening to a patient to use teleconsultation instead of their own clinical judgment to manage the clinical problem. We believe a teleconsultation should have clear aims and objectives to determine why it is happening and exactly what the referring and consulting clinicians are expecting to achieve from it. Common clinical aims for teleconsultations are shown in Table 6.2.

The aims of the teleconsultation listed above in Table 6.2 demonstrate a transition of the primary responsibility of care for the patient from the

Table 6.1   Common Legal Considerations for a Telehealth Program

- Are there any licensure considerations relating to how clinical responsibility is apportioned between the practitioner at the remote consulting site and the advisor at the specialist center?
- What reimbursement mechanisms and contract agreements are needed to ensure payment is made for telehealth services provided?
- Does any of the telehealth equipment used to provide services need to conform to medical devices legislation?
- What is the relationship between the telehealth program and the telecommunications carrier, particularly in respect of any break in service and its speed of restitution and associated compensation?
- Does the telehealth program need to take out a clinical indemnity policy as well as standard insurance cover?
- Are there licensure considerations that relate to work in different countries and/or different states?
- How will privacy and confidentiality regulations be met?

referring clinician toward the specialist clinician giving advice. The process of transferring this clinical responsibility should be formalized wherever possible by incorporating into clear protocols/guidelines. These protocols/guidelines need devising for teleconsultations in all areas of telehealth. When any degree of responsibility for care is transferred between clinicians in a teleconsultation this must be clearly communicated to the patients and/or to their relative/caregiver. For example, in a telepsychiatry consultation a remote clinician may be implicitly seeking advice about the suicide risk of a patient when asking for advice and help in the management of a depressed patient. If the telepsychiatry consultant at the specialist center believes it is appropriate and safe to access the suicide risk of a patient remotely this should be explicitly recorded in a protocol. The protocol/guideline must also specify the requirements for recording information about a teleconsultation. We advise remote sites and specialist centers both keep records of all teleconsultations. Some suggestions for the minimum data set required for a general record are listed in Table 6.3.

The precise records a telehealth program needs to keep for its teleconsultations depends on the clinical area, the practice of individual clinicians, their own standard conventions and good clinical risk management advice. The reason for insisting on a minimum data set for the record is as a way of demonstrating the clinicians at both ends of a teleconsultation have properly discharged their duty of care for the patient. Record keeping in telehealth will become easier with a fully integrated patient record. Unfortunately, this still remains a long way off at present. Record keeping in conventional practice is frequently a major area of unrecognized clinical risk for a health care organization.

Table 6.2   Clinical Aims of a Teleconsultation

- To get factual advice about a technical aspect of care or treatment
- To ask for a second opinion or a corroborative opinion in relation to a course of action recommended for a patient
- To help make an exact diagnosis or differential diagnosis on the basis of a clinical history, clinical examination, and investigations
- To ask for a recommendation about how best to treat a patient and what that treatment should consist of
- To ask advice on the appropriateness of transfer of a patient for care elsewhere and how this transfer should be most safely accomplished

A currently contentious area of record keeping in telehealth is deciding whether or not to videotape a teleconsultation. A video record can be helpful because it authenticates the care took place and for teaching and research. It can also act as a "smoking gun" to indicate possible negligence.[147] In many countries the videotaping of a teleconsultation requires the consent of patients and for this to be formally recorded. Teleconsultations are usually only one part of a wider process of care. Taken out of proper context a videotaped teleconsultation may misrepresent the process of care, or it may clearly illustrate what has taken place. A big consideration when deciding whether or not to record teleconsultations is how to manage the logistics of this process. A person must be assigned to ensure blank tapes are available and then label and archive these tapes after they are full. Because the legal status of these videotapes as medical records is uncertain, how long must they then be kept? An analogous area where this happens is the videorecording of surgical operations particularly when an operating microscope or laparoscope is used. Each telehealth program must decide for itself whether the benefits of recording their teleconsultations make it worthwhile. In doing so they need to weigh up the pros and cons relevant to their own situation, including the cost.

What Reimbursement Mechanisms and Contract Agreements Are Needed to Ensure Payment Is Made for Any Telehealth Services Provided?

The long-term future of telehealth depends on telehealth programs bringing in enough income to sustain themselves. A considerable capital investment is usually needed to establish the infrastructure to support a telehealth program. Clear, contractually secure revenue streams need identifying before any initial investment decisions are made. Health care purchasers usually hold the purse strings to fund new health care projects. They may view

Table 6.3   Suggested Minimum Data Record for Teleconsultations

- Patient name and identifiers, e.g., date of birth, address, social security/NHS number
- Date, time, and duration of consultation, and who participated
- Clear reasons why the consultation was initiated and what were its objectives
- Agreed and disputed findings in the history and examination
- The recommendations as a result of the teleconsultation, any clinical responsibilities assigned, and what was communicated to the patient
- Whether both sides and the patient were satisfied with the process and outcome of the consultation; if not, why not?

teleconsultation with considerable apprehension. These purchasers have already listened to promises of how telehealth will deliver cost savings and make health care more efficient. They have watched the grant funding for telemedicine programs reach an end and have seen the programs unable to finance their future by recouping these promised savings. Currently, health care purchasers' main dilemma is whether to bite the bullet and pay directly for teleconsultations on a fee-for-service basis. The main result they want to see from reimbursing telehealth services is a substitution of this for more expensive forms of face-to-face health care delivery. Purchasers sense a real danger of telehealth consultations substituting for current telephone consultations instead. If this happens, the effect will be their having to pay more to reimburse for telephone consultations they are not currently charged for, and so telehealth will further add to health care cost inflation instead of reducing it.

The United Kingdom has a capitated system of purchasing and providing for health care services. This offers purchasers a simple mechanism to fund telehealth activity in National Health Service (NHS) and reimburse health care providers. Essentially, they can leave it up to the providers to find the solution. If providers can introduce telehealth and stay within their capitated funding they can go ahead. Changes in the NHS and in its contractual arrangements make it important for a telehealth provider outside the NHS to examine any proposed contract carefully and ensure they are protected in the eventuality of health care organizations in the NHS merging. In the United States the situation is more complex. The Health Care Financing Administration (HCFA) is the custodian of the Medicare system and the Medicare trust fund that is currently projected to run out of resources in the early part of the 21st century. HCFA has looked to telehealth to help in providing health care to rural underserved areas and improve the general efficiency of health care. It does not want telehealth activity to become an unnecessary drain on its funds. According to telehealth proponents, a feasible system to reimburse for telehealth requires HCFA to amend its regulations for reimbursement, such as the restriction on physicians being able to jointly bill for a consultation. The definitive results of a 3-year study of tele-health reimbursement begun by HCFA in 1996 are awaited and may help clarify these issues. Summary statistics for HCFA's five-site telemedicine reimbursement study up until 1997 are shown in Table 6.4.

Most notable from these 1997 data is the lack of claims for reimbursement from HCFA for telemedicine services. This finding is significant for two reasons. First, it suggests there is generally low interest in telehealth activity. Second, the protocols for the study show just how seriously health purchasers view telehealth's potential ability to game reimbursement systems.

There is one area for which telehealth reimbursement is now legally provided. In 1997 Section 4206 of the US budget bill was passed and it obliges the US Department of Health and Human Services to reimburse for telemedicine services by January 1999 for Part B of Medicare. Section 4207 of the same bill stipulates a demonstration project is established using "eligible health care provider telemedicine networks" to improve the standard of care for diabetics receiving Medicare in rural underserved or medically underserved inner city areas of the United States. Section 4206 needs to resolve issues of provider payment, noninclusion of telephone line fees or facility costs and the inclusion of coinsurance and deductibles. Section 4207 requires telehealth to link to diabetic care guidelines, assist with diabetic home care, create telemedicine and medical informatics standards and establish a model for the cost-effective delivery of care in both managed care and fee-for-service settings.

The way HCFA is looking at telehealth reimbursement in the United States may seem remote from telehealth programs in the United Kingdom and elsewhere in the world; however, it is important to follow this initiative very closely. Legal changes in reimbursement for telehealth could radically change the future opportunities to expand telehealth services. These opportunities are not being given to telehealth providers on a plate. The dilemmas faced by HCFA over telehealth reimbursement are intrinsically the same as those in all other health care systems. The answers HCFA finds are likely to be replicated in solutions elsewhere. A close watch on this type of initiative will help indicate where potential sources of revenue for telehealth may lie in the near future.

Does Any of the Telehealth Equipment Used to Provide Services Need to Conform to Standards for Medical Devices from Other Regulatory Bodies?

Many items of equipment used in health care must conform to regulatory codes enforced by government bodies such as the Medical Devices Agency

Table 6.4   1997 HCFA Reimbursement Study Claims Figures

CPT Code	IA	NC	WV	Total
99212	—	—	11	11
99213	2	—	—	2
99214	1	—	1	2
99223	—	—	1	1
99231	2	—	—	2
99233	—	—	1	1
99241	1	4	4	9
99242	—	6	1	7
99243	—	2	1	3
99144	1	1	—	2
99251	1	—	5	6
99252	—	—	1	1
99253	12	—	—	12
99254	3	—	—	3
Total	23	13	26	62

From W. England, personal communication, 1998.

(MDA) in the United Kingdom and the Food and Drug Administration (FDA) in the United States. These bodies impose specific standards for the specification, manufacturing standards and uses for health care equipment. Telehealth uses recognized medical devices as well as equipment not previously associated with health care to deliver services to patients. Innovative new ways of delivering health care services raise new issues about the safety of equipment. Telehealth programs must make themselves aware of the regulatory barriers governing the equipment they use to establish any new area of service.

Examples of possible regulatory issues to consider are shown in Table 6.5. These are illustrative examples and not intended as an exhaustive list. It is vital that telehealth programs assess the legal and regulatory aspects well in advance instead of facing the risk of a fine or being shut-down for non-compliance with local, state, or national regulations.

What Is the Relationship Between the Telehealth Program and the Telecommunications Carrier, Particularly with Respect to Any Break in Service and Its Restitution?

A crucial relationship for any telehealth service provider is the one with its telecommunications carrier. Does the duty of care and contractual obligation of a telehealth provider include responsibility to deliver an alternative service in the event of a break in service caused by a failure of the telecommunications carrier? Does the telehealth provider have a standard commercial

Table 6.5   Illustrative Examples of Regulatory Issues Affecting Telehealth

• Specifications for telesurgery equipment in relation to anesthetic gases and electrical conductivity
• Standards of patient monitoring equipment for tele–home care
• Data protection legislation, patient data confidentiality
• Prescribing of medicines using telehealth
• Height of keyboards in workstations, relation to repetitive strain injury
• Health care premises regulations when establishing teleconsultation suites
• Regulations for the storage and disposal of hazardous substances when developing a remote telepathology center

contract to provide services with the telecommunications carrier? The health care industry is becoming dependent on telecommunications systems not only for telehealth but also for data transfer, exchange of health records, referral requests, and clinic bookings. The day-to-day business of health care is becoming intricately bound to the umbilical cord of its telecommunications provider. What standards can a health care provider reasonably expect of services from a telecommunications company? Delays in the installation of Integrated Services Digital Network (ISDN) or T1 lines can be inconvenient and costly for an individual.[148] Delays in ISDN/T1 installation can have profound consequences on the roll-out of a telehealth program. When this happens, losses in terms of both credibility and money can be considerable. A large telehealth program intending to place a sizable contract for telecommunications services usually has considerable leverage in getting a telecommunications company to deliver on time. Smaller telehealth projects with less influence can find this a major source of frustration unless they consider this potential problem well in advance of establishing a service. A major dilemma is that even being a large customer is no guarantee of prompt and efficient treatment by some telecommunications companies.

The legal liability of a telecommunications carrier in the event of a litigation claim associated with delivering telehealth services is a gray area. If the communication channel on which a telehealth service depends fails during a teleconsultation (e.g., during a remote telepresence operation) where does the responsibility lie? Is it the responsibility of the telehealth program to ensure there are fail-safe procedures in case of a breakdown in a communication channel? If there is a prolonged breakdown in the communications channel, can the telehealth program claim for loss of revenue or for the costs of running a substitute service? The situation and potential legal liabilities vary in different parts of the world and need to be investigated. The contractual arrangement a telehealth program makes with a telecommunications company must include these risk management considerations. The lesson to draw from looking at these uncharted waters is for a telehealth program to try to stipulate whenever possible the specifics of its arrangements with its telecommunication carriers in a detailed service-level agreement that reflects the situation of the health care business.

Does the Telehealth Program Need to Take Out a Clinical Indemnity Policy as Well as Standard Insurance Cover?

As with so many other legal aspects of telehealth, this is unclear, and it varies from country to country. Each telehealth program must consider its own position carefully and take legal and indemnity insurance advice. Telehealth activity usually takes place at the interface between health care provider organizations and in high-risk situations such as emergency care, where litigation is extremely common. Telehealth programs must look at all their clinical activities to assess whether an appreciable risk of a clinical negligence claim exists. Aspects of clinical risk face all telehealth providers. The level of risk they face depends on factors such as those shown in Table 6.6.

A decision about whether to take clinical indemnity cover and if so at what level of premium is a business decision for the board of a telehealth program. The board must act on financial risk management advice from the chief financial officer and a clinical risk management assessment of its own organization's clinical activity as well as one of its actual and potential clients. When telehealth is a department within an organization, clinical indemnity questions can be ignored and the dangerous assumption made that these are covered under the umbrella of the whole organization. Does a telehealth organization have a duty of care to its customers, who are ultimately the patients, or do these considerations rest with the clinicians? Does a duty of care include providing means of financial redress in case of a clinical incident? Telehealth programs commonly interpret these questions in a variety of ways. This is reasonable because the scope of clinical activities undertaken by telehealth programs varies, as do their relationships with other health care providers. Whatever eventual decisions are made, these are issues of which the board of a telehealth program must be made aware.

The reason for this board awareness is pragmatic, not to interfere in an operational matter. The legal damages/settlement costs of a major negligence claim against a telehealth organization is a major area of possible financial risk. As such it must feature in the business plan. Even if a telehealth company only acts as a facilities management service to provide telehealth transactions and leaves the responsibility for clinical care with a health care organization, this area still needs clarification.

Table 6.6   Factors that Affect the Clinical Risk of Telehealth Programs

- Whether the telehealth program is predominantly a facilities management company for teleconsultation or a health care provider
- The type of clinical activity being performed
- The s' ills and competencies of the practitioners
- The presence of a clinical risk management program
- The presence of clinical guidelines and protocols
- A clinical audit program
- The level of litigation in the patient population the telehealth service serves

Do Licensure Considerations Exist That Relate to Telehealth Activity with Different Countries and/or Different States?

Telehealth programs must consider the possible legal ramifications of who uses their system to provide health care services as well as the level of health care provided. Legal barriers exist which prevent free mobility of doctors to practice exist in different countries, states, or provinces. Telehealth programs can find themselves in a virtual no-man's-land in terms of the legality of doctors to practice if they are not careful. The United Kingdom and the European Economic Community (EEC) have free mobility of doctors who have acquired the prerequisite qualifications to practice in any other EEC country at the same professional level. This situation is not the same everywhere.

In the United States the situation is much more confused. Each state is responsible for the licensing of doctors to practice within its geographical boundaries. The current situation is outlined in the 1998 Compendium of Telemedicine Laws.[149] This details many of the legal requirements that telehealth providers must meet if they intend to provide services across state lines in the United States.

THE MEDICOPOLITICAL ARENA SURROUNDING TELEHEALTH LEGISLATION AND REGULATION

Many people interested in telehealth and anxious to see it progress are frustrated when they hear that the legal framework it operates in is so vague. Telehealth will radically change how health care is delivered in the 21st century. As telehealth brings about these changes, it also raises political, social, economic, professional, and consumer issues to be addressed. The process of resolving these issues will provide the clear legal framework around telehealth activity. We cannot predict exactly what this framework will be, but we can identify some issues that will influence it and look at how various scenarios may play out. We know the changes telehealth will bring to health care will not be neutral. There will be winners and losers. The main contenders who are currently engaged in the medicopolitical wrestling affecting telehealth legislation and regulation include

- Professional organizations in health care
- Government
- Telecommunications companies

Telehealth is not a topical issue concerning patients and consumer groups in health care.

Neither professional organizations nor the health care professionals within them should imagine they will be left alone to decide the future of telehealth in countries like the United States and the United Kingdom. Throughout the 20th century, governments have intervened to guide and influence the relationship between patients and practitioners. They have done this primarily by introducing regulation and legislation to create frameworks for developing and maintaining professional standards in health care. Frameworks like these can quickly become trade barriers that affect health care delivery both within and between countries. In the United Kingdom, where over 80% of health care activity is publicly funded, and in the United States, where 50% is publicly funded, governments will want their say in what happens to telehealth.

Before looking at how the interplay of interest between outside groups and government influences telehealth, it is worth pointing out how the traditional freedom that governments have had to make decisions is being curtailed with the move to global markets. Health care is a notable exception to this recent trend toward globalization in whole sectors of commerce and industry. Paradoxically, telehealth may play a part in leading sectors within the health care industry to follow a similar global path. If this does happen, what might it mean for professional organizations in health care? An example of the unexpected effect of the North American Free Trade Agreement (NAFTA) for commercial trade is that it undermined the previous profitability of corn-broom manufacturers throughout the United States. Until NAFTA was in place, tariff barriers masked the fact that the product could be produced more cheaply in Mexico. Is it possible that further expansion of the international market for the teleradiological reporting of CT, MRI, ultrasound, and x-rays may similarly affect the salaries of radiologists and the profitability of health care organizations in the United

States? Telehealth and a global market for health care could alter every aspect of how we receive our health care services in the future. Will telehealth spur health care to join the current wave of deregulation, or will it stimulate a rush of protectionism?

The wealthier countries, with their complex health care systems, usually pay physicians the most and raise the greatest barriers to the mobility of doctors. Poorer countries, with a greater need for health care services, put up lower barriers. Telehealth may open up a global marketplace for certain sectors of the health care market. These global markets for telehealth can be realized only if international regulatory and legislative frameworks adapt to accommodate a greater mobility of health care expertise. Mechanisms for setting and maintaining professional standards must then begin to conform within and among countries if this mobility of labor is to occur. Previous national regulation and legislation of physicians in the United States and the United Kingdom have resulted in an unfortunate anomaly. They have centered on the training and educational standards of health care professionals without objectively measuring the "product" they ultimately produce, a product equating to improvement in patients' health. These health benefits result directly from treatment by health professionals. If global products in health care are the future for telehealth, we predict that they will be based on how these products demonstrably affect the health outcomes for individuals in the population and not of a fee-for-service free-for-all.

How the Regulative and Legislative Role of Government May Affect Telehealth

Despite the current fashion for free markets and globalization, government regulators and legislators remain alive and well and surprisingly active. Any review of the legislative programs enacted by the US Congress and UK Parliament confirms their involvement with issues that affect even the minutiae of our daily lives. The eventual substance of these various legislative programs often emerge after gladiatorial tussles have taken place behind the scenes between government and lobbyists from special interest groups. There are already strong interests in the United States and the United Kingdom facing off to influence how telehealth is legislated and regulated. These interested parties include

- Medical and professional organizations
- Pharmaceutical companies
- Medical equipment suppliers
- Telecommunications companies

+ Information technology (IT) equipment suppliers
+ Hospital groups

Industries and organizations throughout the United States and the United Kingdom know they have to involve government in their expansion plans or suffer as a direct result. A recent example was Microsoft Corporation. Microsoft had previously abided by what seemed free-market principles and successfully produced PC software in a highly competitive environment. Their approach to lobbying government had been low-key, generally trying to influence their market environment, such as by objecting to taxation on the Internet. In late 1997, US Attorney General Janet Reno filed a suit against Microsoft on behalf of the federal government to force it to change its policy on selling Internet browsers as part of its core Windows 95 product. Prior to this antitrust assault, Microsoft employed one lobbyist in Washington. Following this legal action the number of lobbyists was increased to three.[150]

Sometimes the economic and political strength of a powerful interest group weighs more heavily than principle in determining the behavior of government. For a long time the tobacco lobby was able to influence politics and economics to prevail over public health issues. Few of us can afford to be critical or cynical about the process of lobbying government for self-interest. Many of us belong to an interest group of one kind or another. Seventy percent of people in the United States belong to an association of some kind, and 40% belong to four or more organizations.[151] Lobbying is now an accepted part of the legislative process.

Government regulation and legislation will seriously affect the future growth potential of telehealth services. The complexion that any eventual legislation takes on is not a random process. Legislation in telehealth is emerging from hard-fought battles involving the clash of committed forces with strong vested interests, both in the development and in the obstruction of telehealth. Entrepreneurial organizations that are directly involved in telehealth or intend to use telehealth to cement their market advantage in other areas are actively looking at the different business scenarios that legislation and regulation may present them. Whether or not they are actively lobbying now, most are watching the legislative process very carefully. They want to be the first off the starting blocks, not left standing when changes to policy, regulation, or legislation occur to affect the market for telehealth. Some changes in this market are predictable; others are still hanging in the balance. Who are the likely power brokers and what regulatory and legislative changes should we look for that will make a difference to the future of telehealth?

The Medical Lobby and Medical Licensure on Telehealth

Medical professional organizations are powerful lobbying forces to which governments usually pay close attention. They pay attention because health is an important political issue and because these organizations expend large amounts of time, energy, and money in lobbying. Medical professional organizations usually combine being very good at lobbying with being discreet. Few of them have publicly stated a definitive position on telehealth. Telehealth poses a real dilemma for the medical establishment of many countries. Although telehealth promises to reduce the costs of health care and expand health care coverage, professional organizations are concerned that this may have adverse effects on their members, including reduced employment of doctors and income reductions. National medical organizations receive the bulk of their income from membership. They therefore represent the interests of their constituent doctors. This position can create conflicts for them when changes to the delivery of health care services, such as telehealth, are proposed.

Given this background status quo, how should we predict that a national medical organization representing dermatologists in Los Angeles or London would react if these physicians faced a competitive threat from a rival group of dermatologists teleconsulting from Vienna, Austria? We would expect these medical organizations to raise major objections. They would cite differing standards of care, continuity of care, medicolegal questions, and a threat to the livelihood of their members as some of the problems. Does this attitude make sense from the perspective of an ordinary patient with a skin complaint? If a patient of these same threatened dermatologists were to visit Vienna on holiday, she/he could receive advice from the Viennese dermatologists without any objection.

By creating new possibilities for how health care is delivered, telehealth inevitably raises awkward questions about the cost, quality, and equity of existing health care delivery systems. Medical organizations are naturally protective of the medicopolitical status quo in these tricky situations. Their general membership fears that the technology will bring with it competition from big health care providers.[152] Are these protective instincts valid responses? Will we as consumers of health care risk losing something valuable if we are not protected from ourselves? The Luddites objected to the mechanization of agriculture on similar grounds yet were eventually overwhelmed by the pressure of the economic force against them. Should medical protectionism block the development of telehealth nationally and internationally? If it can, is this justifiable? Is it tolerable in the face of the difficulties countries have in providing adequate health care to their populations?

Medical Licensure As a Legislative Barrier to the Expansion of Telehealth

National politics and differing legislative processes affect how medical licensing and accreditation varies from country to country and also within individual countries. Physician groups are territorial in nature and usually establish representational structures at hospital, city, regional, and national levels. Differing dynamics exist between medical organizations and legislatures. This creates interesting international differentials in the licensing and accreditation of doctors to practice using telehealth. These differences may be a major medium-term factor determining the relative uptakes of telehealth in different parts of the world.

In the United States the most important aspect of how this dynamic governs the development of telehealth occurs at the interface between the medical lobby and the legislative process at an individual state level. It is here that medical licensure is a major impediment to the growth of telehealth.[153] Each of the 50 states and the District of Columbia manages medical licensure of doctors in its geographical boundaries in conjunction with its state medical board. One function of these boards is deciding the exact licensure requirements for doctors using telehealth systems. The Federation of State Medical Boards (their national association) produced a Model Act to help states in formulating how to grant limited telemedicine licenses to physicians. No state has adopted this Model Act so far. California agreed to let out-of-state doctors practice using telemedicine but only in consultation with a California-licensed physician.[154] States' regulations are continually changing. Many sites on the Internet have current information.[154]

These licensing deliberations are crucially important in influencing the decisions of doctors who are considering joining a telehealth program. If a doctor practices medicine and uses telehealth without complying with state licensure requirements she/he risks loss of insurance coverage, criminal or civil litigation, and Medicare debarment. The sheer logistics and out-of-pocket expense for doctors of obtaining and then maintaining multistate licensure is a major block to the growth of widespread telehealth activity. How future decisions about licensure for telehealth will play out at the individual state level may be a major limitation on the rate of growth of telehealth services on the provider side of the health care system.

Medical licensure limitations on the practice of telehealth create problems for purchasers, such as health payment plans and health maintenance organizations (HMOs) interested in implementing telehealth solutions. Patients of health plans and HMOs sometimes find it more convenient to cross a state line and go to a hospital in an adjacent state. Reducing the costs associated with travel and delays in diagnosis and treatment make telehealth an attractive option for these payers to consider. Paradoxically, they find that most states bar patients who travel across a state line and physically see physicians from making exactly the same consultation from within their own states using telehealth. These seemingly contradictory circumstances limit the health plan/HMO to introducing telehealth only within a state. For some patients this would mean changing the traditional patterns in referral of patients to hospitals. Instead of using the nearest hospital, which might be just across the state line, telehealth would mean linking to a more distant hospital within the same state boundary. If, after the teleconsultation, the patient needs transfer to a hospital, continuity of care would involve traveling a greater distance to an unfamiliar hospital in the same state, one that relatives and friends may find inconvenient to visit. Convenience aside, there are two commercial implications for a health plan: (1) patients may perceive telehealth as taking away their choice and so may choose to change health plans, and (2) increased travel costs (e.g., longer ambulance journeys) may force health plans to raise premiums. In this uncertain environment, one in which the access to specialist services in other states is often effectively blocked, many health plans and HMOs view telehealth as an unnecessarily risky investment, one in which there is little prospect of either generating extra income or finding cost savings to justify it. Although we understand the fears of physicians who have incomes to protect, we also see the illogicality of this in a system where cost disenfranchises so many people from the health care they need.

In the United Kingdom and most of Western Europe the medical licensure and accreditation situation facing health care providers and purchasers considering adopting telehealth is very different. In Europe, telehealth has fortuitously coincided with the creation of a single market for doctors throughout the European Economic Community (EEC). As of 1997 any trained doctor is free to work throughout the EEC; there is a register of all specialists who have completed a training program approved by the EEC countries. A trained dermatologist from Florence, Italy, can therefore theoretically practice in Cardiff, Crete, or Cologne providing she/he can find work. This freedom of medical practice was not prompted as an enlightened proposal by national medical organizations. It came as a by-product of other EEC regulations. When the EEC sought reciprocal recognition of professional qualifications as part of laws intended to enable labor mobility, physicians were rolled in and could not be excluded as a special case. Consequently, there are effectively no similar regulatory and legislative barriers associated with medical licensure and accreditation to prevent open teleconsultation throughout the EEC.

What do these diverse approaches to medical licensing and accreditation mean for the development of telehealth in the near future? The medical lobby is a powerful force, yet recent experience in Europe suggests it will bow to economic forces from outside when these are stronger. From a wider societal perspective the general economy supports the health care system. There now seems to be growing realization by professional organizations that governments and voters view threats to the general economy as taking precedence over parochial medical issues. When approached in the right way, the medical lobby does change. Understandably, winning changes means finding formulas that are acceptable and positive for physicians. The health professions can fear telehealth but should weigh this fear against the many positive economic attractions a global market for telehealth services may bring. They also have to consider what may be the opportunity costs of not taking part in this development. Although there are still language, legal, and logistical issues to resolve, there is now a free market for medical labor in the EEC, one that encourages the growth of telehealth internationally. In the United States many health care organizations are happy about the use of telehealth to penetrate lucrative health care markets overseas (e.g., in the Middle East, Asia, and Europe) yet at the same time want to protect their own health care market. Patchy international telehealth activity is occurring. Will further development of this be blocked in some countries (e.g., the United States) by barriers created by licensure of practitioners? Will the licensure restrictions to telehealth in the United States help to preserve a fragile health care system under threat or cause it to lose out on efficiency gains happening elsewhere? Ultimately, the market will decide which it is to be.

THE HEALTH CARE CONSUMER AS AN ECONOMIC AND POLITICAL PRESSURE GROUP

So far, consumer pressure is an unknown quantity in deciding the future of telehealth. The uptake of health information sites on the Internet adds an interesting and rapidly evolving new dimension to telehealth. The United States has over 40 million people who are uninsured and are limited in their ability to access formal health care. Paradoxically, the richest country in the world has people in a position similar to those in some developing countries in that both groups lack adequate access to basic health care services. Governments are having a difficult time in regulating the Internet. Directly taxing goods and services sold on the Internet is complex. How do you tax the situation where a jacket made in California is sold in Scunthorpe and delivered by an international carrier? If you can tax this transaction, where does the revenue go? Medical advice is now being dispensed from a variety of Internet sites and in some cases appears to blatantly disregard local and national licensure. If health care delivery via the Internet grows, how will this be regulated? If it is regulated, how can such regulations be enforced? Telehealth has not yet excited health care consumers in relation to how they receive care. When it does, we predict that consumer pressure will be the single most powerful force directing the future of telehealth and that this will be Internet-driven. Government attempts at regulation and taxation of the Internet will be a key factor to watch as this develops.

THE TELECOMMUNICATIONS LOBBY AND LEGISLATION FOR TELEHEALTH

Telecommunications companies are major lobbyists of governments, and they are heard. Many governments have to tread a difficult path in telecommunications regulation and legislation. New Zealand, the United Kingdom, and the United States chose early deregulation of their telecommunications industries to stimulate competition and reduce costs. Other countries are now following this example. In deregulating telecommunications, governments expect the competitive environment to be the catalyst that reduces costs and expands network capacity. This strategy is aimed at developing the underlying infrastructure investment in the information age from private capital and not through government spending. To stimulate a fertile financial climate to attract private capital, governments have to find a balance between offering incentives for telecommunications companies to invest and taxing revenues to prevent runaway profits. Being realistic, telehealth is not currently seen within government or the telecommunications industry as a major target for investment. Commerce, training, and education all have higher priorities.

Although telehealth is not a major item in most governments' telecommunications strategies, when viewed in terms of monetary investment rather than words, it does feature strongly in their future thinking. Telehealth is now commercially feasible because of recent technological developments in the telecommunications industry; however, views about the future commercial viability of telehealth are mixed.[155] Telecommunications companies and health care organizations have begun to form quasi-commercial relationships to develop telehealth but have not come up with the magic formula to generate the scales of revenue generation needed to take it higher in the agenda of government or shareholders. The interest of telecommunications companies in telehealth is currently developmental rather than commercial.

Telecommunications companies are taking a "wait and see" approach, a stance that many visionaries who regularly enunciate the future prospects for telehealth find immensely frustrating. The harsh reality of political life is that telehealth has not yet proved it has enough commercial clout to be worth lobbying for by telecommunications companies. It therefore takes a poor second place to education in most governments' telecommunications priorities.

Most telecommunications companies are clearly interested in the potential market for telehealth products and sales of bandwidth. What they are unclear about is the relationship telehealth should have to their core business activities. Many telecommunications companies are going through a midlife crisis about who they are, what they are, and where they are. They are uncertain about what their core business is and what it should be in the future. This crisis of confidence arises from fears that the commercial future of telecommunications companies as simple carriers of information is now almost time-expired. Many fear a future scenario where almost unlimited bandwidth at almost zero cost prevails in the market. If so, profit margins will drastically fall, and many of the current players will be in jeopardy. This scenario predicts that either smaller numbers of carriers with immense volumes of traffic will survive or that current telecommunications companies will have to diversify and become suppliers of information and services as well as bandwidth to attract new revenue.

Telecommunications companies already have substantial markets in health care, markets in their traditional areas of core business of providing telephone, cellular, and pager services to hospitals and other health care facilities. They are well aware of the potential for market growth in areas such as integrated services digital network (ISDN) and T1 and other digital services for telehealth and transferring data to and from health care organizations. What telecommunications companies agonize over is how much they want to get involved in the health part of the telehealth equation. Cash-strapped health care organizations often see the telecommunications companies less as partners and more as potential wealthy donors. They often don't realize how recent history has made telecommunications companies less avid donors and instead profit seekers who are very keen to reap the rewards of investment.

In the 1990s the investment strategy of several US telecommunications companies was to diversify. As part of this strategy some invested in the UK cable television market. Coming after deregulation they saw this market as a ripe plum ready for the taking, an ideal area in which to diversify. Unfortunately, many got badly burned in the process. Their business plans predicted large profits based on a seemingly reasonable assumption that there would be a 45% uptake of cable by British homes, based on parallel experience of cable uptake in the United States. Instead of large profits, companies reaped dramatic losses. The uptake of cable was only 22%, less than half the predicted level. The companies made several mistakes, the most crucial of which was probably their reliance on treating cable as their product and not giving attention or investment to the content (programming). Their major competitor and the current market leader in the United Kingdom is British Sky Broadcasting (BSB). BSB's diametrically opposite strategy was to concentrate on programming and giving consumers what they wanted from the telecommunications revolution. They purchased the rights to products their market research told them consumers wanted, such as sports events. Satellite television now reaches 4.3 million homes in the United Kingdom; cable has reached only 2.2 million homes.

What have the cable companies been successful in selling to UK homes? Telephone connections. They achieved this by undercutting the prices of their indigenous UK rivals. The lessons learned from this and from similar attempts by nervous and bullish telecommunications companies to diversify is that they must focus on their core competencies and decide on their core business. A reflection of this in the United States is AT&T's sale of the credit card company it founded. AT&T now seems to be concentrating on its core business as a telecommunications company and has purchased TCI. Is it adopting the same approach that Coca-Cola took in the 1990s to reemerge as a successful company—focusing back on the core business in which it established its original success? Coca-Cola rejuvenated itself by selling off non-core assets and concentrating on its strength as a soft drinks manufacturer after its performance faltered as a widely diversified company.

In late 1997 the telecommunications company MCI was hotly courted by British Telecom, Worldcom, and others, finally succumbing to the advances of Worldcom, a chase that reflects another of the strategies for survival of telecommunications companies: offering their home and business consumers a package linking local call networks to long distance and Internet services. These telecommunications companies are seeing themselves as the pipelines of information services into homes and businesses. They are interested only in the programming on these pipelines if they are already well-worked-out packages that generate income easily. This brings us back to telehealth. Telehealth is not currently worked through into easily deliverable packages that telecommunications companies can deliver commercially.

Nonetheless, most telecommunications companies are toying with the idea of offering telehealth services. This poses three major problems for them. First, they still view telehealth as an area of new development and outside their core business. Second, their shareholders want to see growth figures well beyond the returns that an investment in telehealth can currently offer. Third, most telecommunications companies are still managed as hierarchical organizations under distinct product divisions. These product divisions are arranged in separate "silos" that communicate badly with one another. This arrangement is not conducive to collaborating with outside organizations in the way telehealth requires. Working with large telecommunications companies is often a challenging experience because their concept of networking often seems embedded in the fiber the organization lays, not in the way people work together.

A solution to organizational inertia for telecommunications companies is to outsource their telehealth operations. This is happening through commercial alliances and direct investment in telehealth start-up companies. This outsourcing is indicative of the current feeling of telecommunications companies about telehealth. They view it as a significant area for investment, but they don't want to repeat debacles like the cable experience in the United Kingdom. Telehealth is on hold as a major area of investment until the profits are more obviously apparent. In this current scenario we can predict the likely behavior of the telecommunications companies as to how they will lobby government over telehealth. They will lobby to promote telehealth through regulation, legislation, and investment that feed into areas of their current core business activity, areas where they are sure they will see revenue. In the short term the most likely areas will directly relate to their role as simple providers of information pipelines.

In deregulated environments, where the market must decide and government is relatively powerless to intervene directly, frustrated proponents of telehealth frequently rail against government, saying, "they should do something." They are less able to say what it is that government should do. Governments are hampered in how much they can promote any one area of policy no matter how important it is to them, let alone one of lower priority like telehealth. Effectively, government can act only at the level of the market and use regulation and/or financial levers to guide and direct market decisions that organizations make in an intended direction. Decisions that governments make concerning telehealth fit into the wider policy area of health informatics. Both the UK and US governments have made some attempts to stimulate telehealth by trying to intervene in the telecommunications market. Each government has tried different and predictable packages. The US government has offered direct subsidy, and the UK government has offered protective support to develop the infrastructure. How have these policies been implemented and what are the implications for the future growth of telehealth?

The US Government and Telecommunications Subsidies to Encourage a Free Market Approach to Telehealth

The US government has taken the line of trying to stimulate the deregulated market to promote telehealth. The Telecommunications Deregulation Act of 1996 established a Universal Service Program, the intention of which has been to subsidize telecommunications companies to provide telehealth and Internet services to rural areas. The United States has effectively adopted an open systems approach. The intention of the US legislation is to create a telecommunications network that is similar to the Postal Service. Just as the cost of a stamp is the same regardless of whether a letter is being sent from the country or the city, the US legislation is designed to equalize telecommunications costs so as not to be discriminatory against where a person lives in delivering health care. With a large potential market for telehealth in rural areas in the United States, telecommunications subsidies are seen as leveling the playing field and stimulating the growth of services for health care.

The UK Government and Legislation for a Protected Market Approach to Telecommunications for Telehealth

There has been no formal policy on telehealth in the United Kingdom.[82] Strands of a policy exist in a variety of different places. The most important of these from a UK government perspective relates to establishing the National Health Service (NHS) telecommunications network in the mid-1990s. The NHS-wide network is a communications network dedicated to the NHS and available at a charge for clinical, management, research, and information gathering purposes. Telehealth was specifically included within the original request for proposals to deliver this network. The contract was awarded to two British telecommunications companies. The strategy in the United Kingdom presupposed that if government provided the framework (soil), telehealth and other products would self-generate (seeds). The incentives for the telecommunications companies were the initial contract but also the opportunity to develop new business as virtual monopoly suppliers with a protected market for 5 years. What is the experience of this approach for the development of telehealth?

From the perspective of a potential service user trying to develop telehealth, the early results were disappointing. They were what would be anticipated from using a closed systems approach to meet the information technology requirements of an organization as immense and complex as the NHS with a large number of legacy systems. As an organization the NHS was said in the early 1990s to be the second largest employer in Europe after the Soviet army. Both these big organizations have since changed. A flavor of some of the complexities associated with using a large closed systems network in health care are given by the following examples from the NHS.

Some of the large academic hospitals, organizations with the greatest potential use for the network and interest in telehealth, found themselves unable to join the network. They faced major logistical problems in complying with the security requirements stipulated to preserve the confidentiality of patient data. They have needed to create complex firewalls to separate the NHS-wide network from other data systems that were deemed insecure. The most notable of these have been the academic networks and the public Internet, which are not considered secure. The chief executive officers of NHS Trusts (UK health care providers) have to take personal responsibility for data security. They have to give personal assurances that minimum standards of data security are met before they can link to the network.

Firewalls are complex and costly to maintain. Data security is difficult in several hundred large organizations, some of which operate on 22 sites and are spread over 100 square miles. If enthusiastic organizations were early adopters and braved the logistics of joining the network, they faced the "first telephone phenomenon." Of what use is the telephone if only you have one? Not only was it difficult to communicate with other organizations using the NHS-wide network, it was found almost impossible to access the Internet and so risked losing contact with organizations with which they could previously communicate. The savings with IT come if you can change processes. In a vast organization like the NHS, being part-on and part-off, a network imposes costs and inefficiencies in needing to "double run" information technology processes.

Introducing the NHS-wide network as a closed network meant problems for hospitals in having to comply with the security standards. This had an added irony when the network was boycotted by physicians in primary care on the advice of the British Medical Association (BMA). Their concern was about the confidentiality of medical records. The legitimate concerns of the BMA are not the point, but rather the problems of trying to introduce an IT project on the scale of the whole NHS and one with which telehealth is expected to interface. The point of this illustration is to show how complex the issues are in introducing information technology into health care.

Legislation and the Internet As an Open System Solution

Alongside the formal activity of government and dedicated networks sits the Internet. The US government has issued guidelines covering the use of the Internet in the transmission of medical data. One HMO on Long Island is exploring the use of a secure intranet to provide clinical information to doctors.[156] This involves communicating over private links on a local cable network and using SSL (encryption) and Verisign digital certificates. The

Health Care Financing Administration (HCFA) is assessing the use of electronic networks for administrative and health care information and is imminently expected to report on this topic. The open Internet is currently being used in the United Kingdom to transmit store-and-forward type of information for dermatology and pathology despite concerns about patient confidentiality. These early uses of the Internet may pave the way for full-scale telehealth on the Internet. This will require absolutely secure encryption. Regulation of the Internet is a difficult area for governments. The interplay between open systems and closed systems for health care informatics will be a major area to watch, not the least because the costs of IT infrastructure are large investments for health care organizations. Companies investing early have the advantage of a system in place. Companies investing later make savings, incur less capital cost to shoulder, and are more likely to acquire a robust system that actually works.

THE FUTURE OF TELEHEALTH?

In conclusion, after painting a brief picture of some of the interests affecting telehealth, we see a rosy future. The unifying point of contact among government, professional groups in health care, and the telecommunications industry is a focus on consumers. Health professional organizations are rising to the challenge of looking at the outcomes of delivering health care by setting standards for care that relate to patients. The interest of the telecommunications companies is in providing the pipeline for services into the home. Government's concern is to stimulate the information technology infrastructure on which the dawning information age will be based, an infrastructure based on the home.

We can already see a growing alignment of telehealth around the delivery of primary care and preventive health care services to people in their own homes. This is where the high-volume, low-cost formula that has fueled the expansion so many industries have been based on can apply to telehealth. We see the platform for this expansion being an open system such as the Internet, where consumer preference can drive the growth of health care services. The main obstacles to be overcome in making this possible are (1) legislative, to remove trade barriers, and (2) technical, to improve data security. It is not surprising that in the short term a highly regulated industry such as health care faces obstacles in integrating with deregulated telecommunications networks. This will change. It is interesting to see the interest of consumer IT companies in health care on the Internet as a major area of growth potential.

7

The Market for Telehealth Services

The precise size of the telehealth market is unknown but is clearly very large. Telehealth is one aspect of an informatics revolution transforming the way health care is delivered worldwide. The estimated size of this health care informatics market is currently $15 billion per year.[157] This market is in turn part of the $1 trillion per year spending on health care in the United States alone.[158] These figures give an approximate indication of the sheer size of the markets in which telehealth services operate and the potential revenue streams available to tap into. We see the uptake of telehealth in the US health care system as a good indication of the way telehealth markets will develop in the future, for the following reasons:

- The move of the major world focus of telehealth activity to the United States and the huge potential size of the US health care market for telehealth.
- The data available on the amount of telehealth activity taking place in the United States.
- The size of the market for telehealth technology in the United States and the number of high-tech companies involved in developing and refining this technology.
- The number of grant-funded telehealth programs in the United States that are spearheading the future development of telehealth services.
- The economic and social forces for change affecting the US health care system and the opportunities for adopting new telehealth solutions.

The uses for telehealth now reach into all aspects of health care delivery in the United States. The potential size of this telehealth market will grow by hundreds of millions of dollars per year. The level of telemedicine activity in the United States tripled between 1995 and 1996, with especially high utilization by mental health and emergency medicine practitioners.[159] Although total US telemedicine consultation rates doubled between 1996 and 1997, this resulted in an average of only 37.4 consultations per site per year by the top 50 US telemedicine programs surveyed.[159] This data suggests that, despite the extent of interest in telehealth and the amount of investment in this technology, its current impact on the delivery of health care in the United States is infinitesimal. In contrast, over 27 million people receive health care from Medicare alone each year in the United States.[160] Given these data, when is it likely that the market for telehealth will grow to a size where it makes a significant impact on the delivery of health care? In this chapter we look at the changing face of health care delivery and what this means for telehealth. We see two components in the development of telehealth: a preliminary market for telehealth equipment and a parallel market for delivering telehealth services lagging further behind. Some markets are ripe for introducing telehealth because telehealth offers a potential solution to otherwise seemingly insoluble problems associated with delivering health care.

HEALTH CARE SYSTEMS AND MARKETS FOR HEALTH CARE SERVICES

Telehealth services are part of wider markets for the delivery of general health care services. An understanding of the market opportunities for telehealth services is helped by a review of the situations facing health care systems in the United States and the United Kingdom in which telehealth products must be developed and sold. This review offers a perspective on the attitudes of health care systems toward investment in new technology and the likely forces driving or hindering investment in telehealth.

Investment in new technology can be problematical for health care systems in the United States and the United Kingdom. The United States spends double the amount on health care spent by the United Kingdom. It is not clear that this investment contributes to a significant improvement in the health of the US population, as health data from the Organization for Economic Cooperation and Development (OECD) in Table 7.1 show.[161]

Using life expectancy and infant mortality rates as proxy measures for the health of the population shows that the United Kingdom (where half as much of the GDP is spent each year on health care as is spent in the United States):

Table 7.1   Comparative US/UK Health Data and Spending

Measure relating to spending on health care	UK	US
Spending on health care as % of GDP in 1996	6.9%	14.2%
Per capita spending on health care in 1996	$1,304	$3,708
Median age of the population in 1995	37 yr	35 yr
Percentage of the population over 65 years old in 1995	15.8%	12.2%
GDP per capita (adjusted for purchasing power) 1995	$17,923	$25,635
Inpatient hospital beds per 1,000 population in 1995	4.7	4.1
Average length of stay in hospital by patients in 1995	9.9 days	8.0 days
Percentage of the population admitted to hospital in 1995	20.8%	12.4%
Population eligible for public-funded hospital care (1995)	100%	46%
Infant mortality per 1,000 live births (1995)	6.0/1000	8.0/1000
Life expectancy of males at birth (1995)	74.3 yr	72.5 yr
Life expectancy of females at birth (1995)	79.7	79.2

- Has as healthy a population as the United States.
- Has universal health care coverage for the population.
- Admits more people to hospital for longer periods of time than in the United States.

Additional data[161] show how the number of computer tomographic (CT) scanners compares between the two countries. The United Kingdom has 6.3 CT scanners per million people in the population, compared to 26 per million in the United States. The number of magnetic resonance imagers (MRI) was 3.4 per million in the United Kingdom, compared to 15.5 per million in the United States. If the numbers of CT and MRI scanners are taken as proxy figures for each of the countries' expenditures on health care technology, this suggests that the discrepancy in expenditure between the United States and United Kingdom is due, at least in part, to the level of investment in technology.[162]

Whether the health care system is funded publicly or privately, it is an overhead cost to industry within a country. The international free trade agreements now in existence, such as a single market in the European Economic Community and the North American Free Trade Agreement (NAFTA) mean that any increased health care expenditure inevitably feeds through into higher costs of production for industry and higher prices for goods and services. Price rises from funding health care make the goods and services produced by a nation more expensive to sell both at home and abroad.

Because of this any attempt at introducing new technology (e.g., telehealth) into the health care system is now subjected to close scrutiny in the United States and United Kingdom as part of attempts to curb health care cost inflation. The case for a rigorous analysis of health technology spending received even greater momentum with the realization that many health care interventions have no scientific basis to show that they are effective. This disturbing finding damages the credibility of the "science of medicine" and has stimulated a vogue for evidence-based medicine programs in the United Kingdom and Canada, as well as parallel initiatives to assess outcome measures for health care services in the United States.

In summary, the general market for health care services has changed considerably since the early 1990s. Before that time new technologies (e.g., CT and MRI) were introduced relatively unquestioningly into communities.[163] Now, new health care technologies, including telehealth, are expected to undergo evaluation before they are introduced. These evaluations are intended to prove the cost-effectiveness and positive benefits to the health of the population of any new technology. Consequently, sales and marketing strategies for telehealth products should establish certain basic facts such as those shown in Table 7.2 if they are going to persuade the health care market to invest in technology.

1. *Establishing that there are reasons for telehealth services to be used if they are offered:* Not all health care activity is suitable to take place remotely. There may be clinical, cultural, legal, or other good reasons that this cannot happen. It is vital to ensure that practitioners and patients accept a telehealth service before establishing a program. Practitioners and patients must understand the logic for why they are being asked to change the current way they deliver or receive health care and use a telehealth system instead. For example, introducing a mobile telehealth system in a paramedic (ambulance) service to support the management of sick patients in transit to hospital makes clinical sense. Paramedics can communicate ahead to the receiving hospital. The hospital can prepare the emergency room for a sick or injured patient and get advice on how to start lifesaving treatments in advance of his/her arrival at the hospital. However, a telehealth system must make practical as well as clinical sense. Let's return to the same hypothetical ambulance/paramedic situation. Does it make practical sense to install a telehealth system to support paramedics? What if cumbersome equipment takes up half the ambulance space, the data connection is unreliable, and the eventual results of introducing the system don't improve the outcome for patients?

2. *Establishing that there is evidence that a telehealth service saves costs, improves quality, or increases market share for the health care organization*

Table 7.2   Strategies to Sell Telehealth Services in Health Care Markets

---

- Establish that there is a clinical reason to use a telehealth service if it is offered.
- Establish that there is evidence that a telehealth service saves costs, improves quality, or increases market share for the health care organization being approached to buy telehealth services.
- Establish that there is a market for the telehealth service if this is offered.
- Ensure that the telehealth program/company persuades a customer to buy its telehealth services and not the more general idea of buying telehealth services.

---

being approached to buy telehealth services: A telehealth services has to show that it is effective. Does it really improve the care of the patient? If a patient with a skin lesion is seen by a nurse practitioner or by a physician assistant, will the telehealth system enable her/him to get advice from a dermatologist and make a reliable diagnosis in a comparable number of cases to conventional practice methods? If it does provide a comparable or better diagnostic service, is it cost-effective? Will using telehealth enable health care organizations to provide services in areas where they otherwise could not and so increase their market share?

3. *Establishing that there is a market for a telehealth service if it is offered:* Clinicians may be very happy at the prospect of a telehealth service, yet there may be no market for the service. A telehealth service may be prohibitively expensive because of the initial equipment investment or because of the costs of digital data systems, such as microwave or satellite transmission. The management culture in health care organizations may not accept the new technology, or it may have more urgent priorities for investment elsewhere.

4. *Ensuring that a telehealth service provider manages to persuade customers to buy its telehealth services, not just to buy into the general idea of a telehealth service and then go elsewhere to purchase it:* Telehealth programs that do an excellent job of selling the idea of using telehealth to health care organizations can have the frustrating experience of finding these same organizations buying their telehealth service or equipment elsewhere. These unfortunate service providers must find the right balance between giving helpful information and not giving away details from which they could derive commercial benefit. Considerable time and effort are expended in establishing a workable telehealth service: devising equipment specifications, drawing up clinical protocols, implementing the program, and training staff. A difficult transition for telehealth service providers trying to secure their commercial future is learning how to sell and market their product, as distinct from selling the general idea of telehealth. A visit from a prospective customer to see a telehealth facility can interrupt patient care and have considerable opportunity costs in terms of how a small management team

might otherwise spend its time. Often the greatest asset of a telehealth program is not the equipment it uses but the intellectual property contained in how it configures and delivers health care services remotely. To become commercially successful, a telehealth service provider must be aware of its intellectual property and know how to market it successfully and sell it profitably.

Thinking through the four points above helps a telehealth service provider develop realistic sales and marketing strategies for approaching the wider health care market to sell its products. Telehealth acts as a communications tool to facilitate health care delivery. We believe the intrinsic strength of the technology lies in how it builds clinical communication bridges between health care organizations and other related institutions. A useful way to stratify the market opportunities for telehealth is in terms of the following:

- Primary care applications
- Secondary care applications
- Specialist and academic center applications
- Home care applications
- International applications, including medical repatriation
- Military telemedicine

THE MARKET FOR TELEHEALTH
SERVICES IN PRIMARY CARE

We see a very large and so far untapped market for telehealth services in primary care. Telehealth offers decision-support tools to enhance health care consultations and the vast majority of formal health care consultations that take place between physicians and patients in primary care. In the United States the growing movement toward managed care is bringing with it a growing trend to use care primary care physicians as gatekeepers in a way similar to that of the general practitioner in the United Kingdom. In the United Kingdom the general practitioner traditionally has acted as a gatekeeper to control the direct access of patients to more complex and costly specialist care services. In the late 1990s government policy in the United States and United Kingdom has been to explicitly encourage the trend of moving health care services from hospital settings into primary care, for the following reasons:

- It makes health care services more convenient for patients by placing them closer to where the patients live.

* It helps manage the demand for health care services and reduce costs through the gatekeeper function of the primary care physician.[164]
* It promotes a more holistic approach to delivering health care services than the rigid medical model imposed by a health care system driven from large acute care hospital settings.

Experience in the United States suggests that the move to managed care is making the demarcation between primary care physician and specialist physician ever more pronounced. Specialist physicians are now spending less time in primary care, leaving it to primary care physicians to provide general care instead.[165] The major future market for telehealth in primary care lies in providing decision support to primary care physicians who face a constantly expanding scope of practice from this change on the part of specialist physicians. If our prediction is right, what is the rationale for primary care physicians and specialist physicians buying into telehealth for this purpose? The sales strategies outlined earlier in Table 7.2 provide a framework to answer this.

Reasons for Telehealth Services to Be Used in Primary Care If They Are Offered

Acting as gatekeepers in capitated health care systems, such as in some managed care organizations in the United States and in the United Kingdom's National Health Service (NHS), often puts primary care physicians in a difficult position. A primary care physician can face a potentially conflicting role each time she/he sees a patient. One function of the primary care doctor is to be a traditional physician and act on this set of impulses to champion the rights of patients, offering them the "duty of care" their profession demands them to offer. In a capitated care environment physicians also may have to regulate the access of patients to specialist care, working now on the behalf of the wider health care organization that employs them. This can place the primary care physicians in the invidious position of having to ration care for individual patients for the good of the wider population and the financial health of their employers.

Making these judgments can be very difficult because individual patients vary in how they present with disease. The diagnosis can be uncertain, and managing the patient correctly may depend on knowing the nuances of all the treatment choices available. Physicians are less satisfied with their working conditions because of the constraints that managed care places on the care they are able to provide to patients.[166] Although protocols for care can help resolve some of these conflicts, they can also leave the primary care physician in the position of being seen by patients as agents of an outside body seeking to impose restrictions on their choices of doctor and the level of care they receive.

In these instances it can be difficult for primary care physicians to be sure when to refer patients for specialist treatment and when not to refer, particularly when patients are increasingly demanding that health services give them choice and involvement in the decisions they need to make about their care. Telehealth offers a practical solution to these mounting pressures on primary care physicians. It does this by helping them offer choice about treating their patients, involving them in deciding what care they receive, and helping them to access services more easily. Telehealth can achieve this in four ways:

1. It can allow patients to videoconsult with their primary care physician from home, either directly or by E-mail and avoid unnecessary trips to the office.
2. Telehealth services also can allow patients to videoconsult with their primary care physician and a specialist.
3. Telehealth services can make the services of primary care physicians available in rural areas where they are in short supply.
4. Telehealth can provide continuing medical education services to primary care physicians.

Establishing That There Is Evidence That a Telehealth Service Will Save Costs, Improve Quality, or Increase Market Share for the Health Care Organization Being Approached to Buy Telehealth Services in Primary Care

There is a growing experience in the United States and the United Kingdom of using telehealth in all areas of primary care. There is no good evidence in the telemedicine/telehealth literature to show that telehealth is cost-effective and can produce better clinical outcomes in primary care than conventional methods of practice. This does not mean that telehealth does not have an important future role to play in delivering primary care services. It means that there is not yet the evidence to support widespread policy recommendations for a generalized introduction of telehealth into primary care. It also means that there are no fully worked through applications to offer primary care organizations interested in establishing telehealth services. When working in primary care, telehealth service providers are often in the business of being pioneers working on health services development projects. This puts the onus on a telehealth service supplier to work closely with primary care providers and identify with them the applications for telehealth that solve practical problems in delivering health care, applications to justify their investment in telehealth.

Establishing That There Is a Market for the Telehealth Service If It Is Offered

An important initial step in identifying potential areas of primary care as users of telehealth service is to critically examine existing processes for care delivery. This analysis should concentrate on identifying problems associated with access, equity, and cost of currently delivering care. These problems are usually easily apparent because they are what patients complain about most often. They are also problems an appropriate telehealth application can help resolve. The move toward managed care in the United States and locality purchasing in the United Kingdom presents opportunities for introducing telehealth as a tool to help manage services more efficiently and increase the market share of primary health care providers. One such area of opportunity stems from the Medicare revisions in the 1997 Balanced Budget Act and state health care reform initiatives in the United States. Both provide incentives for managed care organizations to expand the range of services they provide in rural areas. In 1995 only 3.9% of people in rural areas (defined as not being adjacent to a metropolitan area and with no city, or a town with less than 2,500 people) were enrolled in a commercial HMO, compared to 33.3% in large metropolitan area.

Expanding their delivery of primary care services into rural areas can pose major logistical problems to managed care organizations. Primary care physicians play a vital role in the process of health care delivery in managed care. There are already problems in recruiting primary care physicians, nurses, and other staff to work in rural areas of the United States.[162] Telehealth offers a way to make expansion of managed care services into rural areas possible and cost-effective. Telehealth can resolve physician staffing problems and at the same time offer patients increased choice of referral to specialist physicians for advice and treatment. A major strategic consideration for managed care organizations as they try to expand their services into rural areas is how to ensure that they have the necessary information technology support to manage any new health care services they deliver. In arranging the necessary data networks and IT requirements to support routine health care delivery in rural areas, managed care organizations usually provide network infrastructures suitable for telehealth to take place in primary health care, using low bandwidth applications.

In contrast to the United States, where the problems with primary care are often in rural areas, primary care in the United Kingdom usually grapples with how it can offer general practitioner services to inner city areas. Since 1995 an emerging problem with primary care in the United Kingdom has been one of how to recruit physicians into inner-city general practice training schemes. With large numbers of elderly inner-city general practitioners imminently due to retire, there are predictions of major problems with staffing inner-city primary care facilities in the near future. This depletion of general practice trainees may be a short-term trend associated with the changing fashion in physician specialty training. A worrying statistic is the 1995 projection for primary care physician numbers in the United Kingdom suggesting that there will be 30% fewer primary care physicians than the NHS requires by the year 2000.[168] Any shortage of primary care physicians can only exacerbate the existing problems of delivering health care services to inner-city areas. The creative use of telehealth is a possible answer to the problem of maintaining health care services in rural parts of the United States and inner-city United Kingdom underserved by primary care physicians. Using nurse practitioners and physician assistants as a solution to this shortage has been actively explored in the United States and United Kingdom and there are possible models established for using them in telehealth.[169,170]

These newly evolving models of primary care include the concept of using primary care resource centers. If these centers are of sufficient size to include a large enough critical mass of health care and other related services they justify including telehealth facilities. Making primary health care resource centers work effectively often requires altering the pattern of health care service delivery, changing the culture in which health care professionals work and winning over the support of the local population that will use the facility.[170] Primary care was often equated with offering low-technology care in the past. New primary care resource centers include many high-tech applications previously associated with hospitals. These centers are ideally suited for establishing services to support disease management programs for the continuing care of patients with chronic diseases. The inclusion of telehealth into these primary care–based disease management programs is a logical progression.

Telehealth fits closely with implementing disease management protocols in primary care because it can connect primary care physicians (general practitioners) directly to patients for the electronic exchange of information. Telehealth promises to support a range of services in primary care, from mundane administrative tasks such as appointment booking to providing health information, screening programs, remote diagnosis, remote monitoring, and remote treatment. Managed care organizations in the United States and locality purchasers of health care in the United Kingdom already see the potential advantages of the "wired" patient. The easiest and most convenient way to make this connection between patient and primary care physician is through the Internet. Data security and confidentiality are current barriers to this, as is getting a critical mass of personal computers (PCs) into homes. Around 60% of homes in the United States have a PC. Consequently, Internet TV may provide the logical technology link for telehealth into the home. The other major practical difficulty in developing home consultation into a routine service is in the cultural change required for patients and doctors to accept this radical departure from tradition. We suspect the logical development of these home telehealth services will take off from the initially more restricted market of telecare at home.

Ensuring That, As a Telehealth Service Provider, Customers Are Persuaded to Buy Primary Care Telehealth Services and Are Not Just Attracted to the General Idea of Buying a Telehealth Service and Then Going Elsewhere to Buy It

Establishing viable primary care health care services based on telehealth involves considerable process reengineering of existing methods of health care delivery and large investment in new information technology systems. This process reengineering will involve radical changes in how primary care organizations function, changes that extend from how practitioners work to making structural alterations in buildings from which services are delivered. Other care systems with which primary health care services have to interface are complex. It is often necessary to adapt a telehealth system to accommodate the care processes involved, not vice versa.

The disparate nature of primary care services makes the main expertise of telehealth service providers who have any substantial experience in primary care one of establishing and managing complex local area networks (LANs). The greatest complexity of these networks usually relates to "people" issues, such as how people and processes link into information technology, rather than the technology itself. Primary health care services usually involve a range of organizations working together in loose collaborative arrangements. These include hospitals, community nurses, social services departments, housing departments, voluntary organizations, and other welfare organizations. Good examples of this interagency work in primary care are child protection and the care of the elderly. A mistake made by organizations offering telehealth services in primary care when they try to sell their services is to make what they do look too easy, giving the impression that all it requires to be successful at telehealth in primary care is to buy the equipment and establish the IT network. Successful telehealth in primary care requires practitioners who are able to work autonomously but adhere to the policies, procedures, and referral networks needed to make telehealth work. This intellectual property linked to the appropriate information technologies is what a telehealth service provider in primary care has to offer and so often gives away free.

THE MARKET FOR TELEHEALTH IN SECONDARY CARE

There is now a very considerable body of experience in providing operational telehealth at the secondary care level. Secondary care organizations sit in a pivotal position between primary care and specialist care in academic tertiary care centers. In the current uncertain climate for health care delivery, acute care general hospitals are often caught up in crisis management and lack the management capacity and resources required for adequately developing telehealth services. Hospitals can feel a sense of threat, even paranoia, associated with telehealth. This sense of threat usually comes from misinformation or lack of knowledge. In the financial climate in which acute care hospitals operate in the United States and the United Kingdom any competent senior executive capable of taking a telehealth project forward is acutely aware of what are deliverables and what are promises and dreams. Because their job future depends on deliverables, the key to marketing telehealth in secondary care is to offer a clear vision and assured deliverables.

Establishing a Reason to Use a Telehealth Service in Secondary Care If It Is Offered

Telehealth inevitably brings change. Hospitals are hierarchical organizations. They are typically resistant to change, and telehealth is only one of the many changes they face at the moment. Working to develop health services using telehealth involves camaraderie. This camaraderie is born of facing rooms of practitioners in hospitals who are initially deeply suspicious of telehealth and who voice vocal and searching reservations about it. We do not believe that telehealth has a separate agenda from the rest of health care. The key to convincing practitioners of the value of telehealth is to make it relevant to a positive future for health care systems where telehealth is seen simply as a tool to facilitate the delivery of health care and solve problems. Clinicians beset by dealing with the current difficulties of delivering health care in a turbulent environment welcome the opportunity to hear about telehealth when

- They can discuss it with somebody who understands the day-to-day business of delivering clinical care to patients.
- Its introduction is aimed at supporting them in the process of delivering health care and improving the care they can give to patients.
- They are not expected to implement it without support.

Any discussion about telehealth with hospital clinicians must take place with thought, planning, tact, and the clear support of the senior management team in the organization. Unfortunately, there is a lot of hype about telehealth. A public relations disaster for the future of telehealth can occur in an organization when a middle-grade manager attends a conference and repeats rhetoric to busy clinicians, promising that telehealth can deliver the undeliverable. Used creatively to solve problems, telehealth can offer practitioners in acute care hospitals practical ways to change the environment in which they work and help them to dictate the direction of change instead of having it imposed on them.

Establishing Evidence That a Telehealth Service Will Save Costs, Improve Quality, or Increase Market Share for Acute Care General Hospitals If They Invest in Telehealth Services

The short answer is that, except for some isolated examples, there is as little scientific evidence to support the use of telehealth as there is for most of the health care delivered in acute care hospitals. How to resolve the delivery of health care based on evidence in a rapidly changing climate of development and a paucity of evidence is complex.[69] In practical terms, telehealth projects in acute care hospitals need evaluations that interface with outcome evaluation programs in the United States and evidence-based medicine initiatives in the United Kingdom.

Establishing a Market for Telehealth Services in Secondary Care

There is a huge potential market for telehealth in secondary care. The argument for the development of this market is somewhat complex to explain because it means that acute care hospitals see the logic of it as a strategic investment for the future and not a reactive response to the present.

In both the United States and the United Kingdom there has been an inexorable trend toward reduced hospital inpatient stays since the early 1980s because of changes in how health care is practiced. As a result of reduced length of hospital stay, numbers of hospital beds have declined. Conclusive opinions about whether there are too many or too few hospital beds are complex to reach, particularly in the United Kingdom. Regardless of the current adequacy of hospital beds, the situation creates practical consequences at the micro level of managing an individual hospital or group of hospitals. The consequences reduce to either attracting more patients through the hospital to fill empty beds or changing the way hospitals deliver health care and so reduce the number of empty beds. In either scenario there is a major role for telehealth. Hospitals are no longer simple "bed factories" and are being forced to change to attract patients.

One way in which telehealth helps acute care hospitals to attract more patients to use its services is by linking a hospital into primary health care telehealth networks. We have already described the rationale for establishing primary health care telehealth networks. Primary care physicians need decision support when referring patients to hospitals. Linking these decision processes together in protocols that include telehealth establishes the concept of metropolitan telehealth networks based around acute care hospitals in a hub-and-spoke arrangement, as shown in Figure 7.1. Telehealth becomes a way to create more referral spokes to support the hospital hub and attract more patients.

In the future the hospital may use the Internet instead of a wide area network (WAN) to link with primary care centers. As well as offering teleconsultation in a range of specialties and training and education to primary care centers, the acute care hospital can offer a range of other virtual services to primary care, including

* Facilities management of information technology systems
* Human resources and payroll
* Finance and accounting
* Clinical audit and research and development
* Service development
* Shared clinical records and multimedia clinical records

In the current climate, hospitals have the overhead costs of empty beds to support without revenue. New primary care centers can be recruited to join the network via the WAN and increase the patient referral base of the hospital. In developing this strategy the acute care hospital intends to attract a greater volume of referrals from primary care to cover its cost base. An alternative strategy for a hospital is to accept that its role will change in the future and therefore to shed unoccupied beds and downsize. In this scenario the hospital adopts a business strategy based on providing a smaller number of highly specialized services on site and giving remote consultation advice to support a larger network, as shown in Figure 7.2.

Ensuring That a Secondary Care Telehealth Service Provider Persuades a Customer to Buy Its Telehealth Services, Not the General Idea of Buying Telehealth Services and Purchasing Elsewhere

The intellectual property of developing metropolitan telehealth networks lies in developing and maintaining a physical network and in managing the process of teleconsultation between secondary care and primary care. The main problem for telehealth providers with expertise in developing metropolitan networks is how they should respond to requests for proposals or tender for new business to support their development. These often require detailed specifications and large amounts of management time with no assurance of then being awarded the contract, amounting to free consultancy work.

Stage 1. Primary Care Local Area Networks

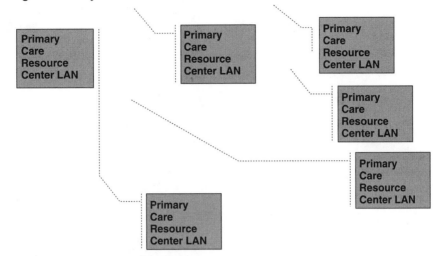

Stage 2. Linking the Hospital LAN to the Primary Care LANs Using a WAN

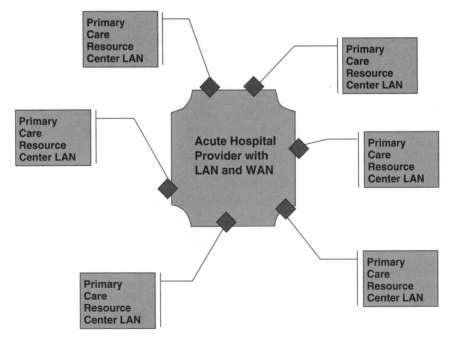

Figure 7.1 Developing a metropolitan telehealth network to increase market share.

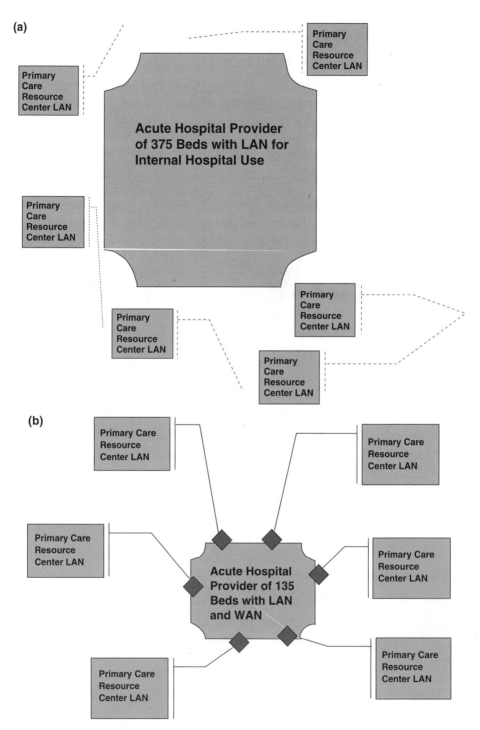

Figure 7.2 (a) A metropolitan telehealth network developed to downsize a hospital before change; (b) metropolitan network with downsized hospital and enlarged primary care centers after change.

THE MARKET FOR TELEHEALTH
IN ACADEMIC MEDICAL CENTERS

Academic medical centers face particular problems because of changes happening in health care systems. In the United States, academic health centers face lost income because of the way managed care organizations and health insurers increasingly negotiate contracts for nonspecialist services. Managed care contracts for these services with general hospitals and so deprives academic health centers of this income. Academic medical centers have supported themselves in the past by providing general as well as specialist medical services, and the loss of this revenue under managed care has led to financial problems. In the United Kingdom, academic centers are trying to survive in relatively unsophisticated health care markets, where the additional costs of research and development and the training and education of health professionals[171,172] are just being taken into account. The cost of support services such as pathology, radiology, hematology, and other general overhead costs contributes to lower income as academic medical centers in the United States and United Kingdom lose revenue. This accounting process makes academic centers' costs greater and prices higher, and they become less competitive. Telehealth offers another way to attract new revenue and prevent the spiral of cost increases from continuing.

Establishing a Reason to Use a Telehealth Service in an Academic Medical Center If It Is Offered

Practitioners in academic centers usually show much the same reluctance toward telehealth as practitioners in acute care general hospitals. Clinicians in academic medical centers are used to having patients referred to them nationally and internationally. These clinicians show particular interest in how they can use telehealth as a way to encourage distant referrals to their specialty and also to help patients avoid unnecessary trips to their institution for investigations and outpatient followup. An area of growing interest to them is how they can use telehealth in research studies. Another area for telehealth, paralleling its clinical care application in many academic medical centers, is the use of teleconferencing for undergraduate and postgraduate teaching.

Establishing Evidence That the Telehealth Service Will Save Costs,
Improve Quality, or Increase Market Share for Academic Medical Centers

There is currently no direct evidence to suggest that telehealth will save costs, improve quality, or increase market share for academic medical centers. Many academic medical centers in the United States have taken the route of using extremely high-cost, high-specification telehealth equipment requiring high bandwidth to operate a service. This decision makes the costs of telehealth in these centers high, and the consultation rates are usually low. This can deny them access to primary care because of equipment incompatibility and high bandwidth requirements. Telehealth can provide patients (and revenue) to academic medical centers, and the business case for each clinical specialty must be clearly established. A sound business case is equally important to showing that telehealth is clinically effective for the development of services in academic medical centers. In the past, reasons such as prestige have often stimulated developments in academic medical centers. In today's health care climate, prestigious developments must usually also pay their way.

Establish a Market for Telehealth Services in Academic Medical Centers If This Is Offered

For reasons similar to those that apply to hospitals in secondary care there is a large market for telehealth services associated with academic medical centers. Academic medical centers have an opportunity to market their expertise more widely by using telehealth. Entrepreneurial centers are actively exploring four markets for telehealth—regional, national, international, and research.

Local health care markets are important for academic medical centers, both in the United States and the United Kingdom. In both countries the hospital sector is downsizing, with a loss of beds, at the same time that primary care services are expanding. The hospital sector (academic medical centers and secondary care) faces two extreme scenarios, with a probability of the final outcome being somewhere between the two. The first scenario is that the secondary care sector increasingly squeezes the academic medical centers into radically restructuring and downsizing themselves to survive. The second scenario is of an alliance between academic medical centers and an expanded primary care sector with a corresponding reduction of general hospitals in the secondary care sector. The intricate details of these scenarios and how they may play out are for another book. From the telehealth perspective what matters is that academic medical centers develop strategies to link into primary care through telehealth networks. If acute care general hospitals in the secondary care sector lock primary care providers into closed metropolitan networks, referrals to academic centers may become increasingly restricted to specialized referral and advice. Economic incentives exist for secondary care providers to manage more specialized cases themselves and refer fewer patients for general care to academic medical centers. The best interests of patients will be served with open networks for telehealth so that patient referral mechanisms are not distorted by restrictions in information flow.

Academic medical centers have the expertise to market regionally and nationally in providing specialist health care services. Patients are already prepared to travel long distances for diagnosis and treatment from an expert center. There are now opportunities for academic medical centers to develop protocols and guidelines for the delivery of care with distant local health care providers with whom they link remotely. The income of the academic medical center becomes less dependent on direct inpatient stays in its own beds and more directed toward the sale of its expertise in remote consultation. The intellectual property on which this specialist advice is based should stem from research done remotely as part of multicenter collaborations. The remote sites delivering care can recruit patients into studies based on protocols for diagnosis and treatment as shown in Figure 7.3.

Academic medical centers with the expertise to market and deliver their health care services regionally and nationally also have the opportunity to sell these services internationally.

Research is a major source of income for academic medical centers. Many centers receive more income from their research activity than from the direct delivery of health care services to patients. In addition to the direct financial effect of lost revenue when purchasers transfer patient care to smaller general hospitals, medical centers face a secondary loss of income from not being able to attract sufficient numbers of patients to make research proposals possible. They are exploring the potential of telehealth to help recruit patients into research studies and maintain this important source of income in two ways.

The first way is to directly link with practitioners in primary and secondary care and attract the referral of patients for treatment and recruitment into their studies. This follows the traditional pathways for patient referral except that it uses technology to sustain a referral network that is shrinking. The volumes of referral to most specialist areas are currently too small to sustain a telehealth network in primary or secondary care of sufficient size to provide a source of referral to research studies. This may become a referral source in the future with the expansion of telehealth networks when there is the volume of usage from routine health care delivery and academic medical centers can tap into them.

The other area academic medical centers are busily exploring is using telehealth as a way of recruiting patients under the care of other providers into multicenter research projects. The Internet works particularly well as a tool for this, with the usual disclaimers about confidentiality of data. The Internet provides a cheap and readily available network to access across the world. Internet database tools, with intranets and extranets, are convenient as data collection tools, posting the template for these data on the Web.

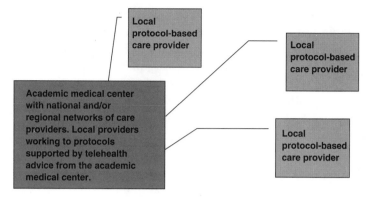

Figure 7.3   National and regional specialist referral networks from academic medical centers.

Practitioners and patients involved in a study can enter data directly, receive updates about the study, and ask questions of the researchers. This data networking simplifies the people and paper processes involved in clinical research and reduce their costs.

We believe that the major growth potential for telehealth by academic health centers will be to provide distributed health care and clinical research services on a large scale in Europe, Asia, and Australia. The United States is a favorable climate for developing most telehealth services but not interstate programs from academic medical centers. Interstate licensure regulations in the United States pose a problem, practically preventing doctors from teleconsulting across state lines. High volumes of referral to specialist centers require large population bases to draw on. Population bases from more than one state are typically required to make specialist telehealth services practicable. The reasons for the medical protectionism that underlie this resistance at a state level are understandable. However, is this ultimately a form of "Luddite" resistance to change? Blocking change in this way may be more damaging than taking the risks of working in new ways and dropping the medical protectionism. The United States health care system has the possibility of leading the world in the development of new health care delivery systems, but it may be forced to watch international initiatives develop in other countries whose health care systems and doctors are prepared to be more innovative.

Ensuring That an Academic Medical Center Buys a Telehealth Service and Not the General Idea of Buying Telehealth Services

Telehealth services connected with academic medical centers are usually complex products to pull together. They require a combination of sophisticated technology and specialist clinicians to run them. The specialist advice center must provide both scheduled consultations and emergency access for remote sites to access. Major logistical issues then come into play. Most academic medical centers run their own telehealth services. They are not always efficiently managed because of a lack of the marketing skills and business acumen needed to run a telehealth program as a commercial venture and not as an outreach clinical research program. Opportunities exist for commercial telehealth companies to set up joint ventures with academic medical centers. Academic centers are usually aware of the potential for telehealth and do not need selling on the idea. The problem academic medical centers and prospective joint venture partners often face is selling the idea of telehealth internally in the organization. Clinicians who find it difficult to come to terms with changes in the delivery of conventional services are difficult to persuade about the advantages of even broader changes such as telehealth.

THE MARKET FOR HOME CARE APPLICATIONS OF TELEHEALTH

With changing demographic profiles in the United States and United Kingdom—an aging population and the reduced time patients spend in hospitals—it is not surprising to find that the fastest-growing section of the health care market in the United States is home care. Medicare spending on home health services increased tenfold between 1987 and 1995, reaching over $17 billion per year.[173] Home care is health care services delivered to people in their own homes. These data are difficult to interpret in the United Kingdom, but the rates of home visits by district nurses and health visitors as recorded by routine activity reports have risen considerably since 1994.[174]

Another important area of home care is the home monitoring of patients. Digital data networks allow patients with illnesses, especially chronic illnesses, to be monitored at home. Monitoring of patients at home enables diagnostic testing to prevent hospital admission, for example, cardiac investigations, diabetic care, and EEGs. It also enables patients to return home earlier from hospital and receive hospice care at home. Early commercial telehealth companies were established in Italy[175] and Israel[176] to provide cardiac monitoring of patients in their own homes.

Establishing that Community Nurses Will Use Tele–Home Care If it Is Introduced

In our experience community nurses are receptive to innovative ideas to improve the care they give to patients. To introduce telecare the working environment of an organization and its culture has to be supportive. Tele–home care cannot totally replace the traditional contact between nurse and patient, but it can make the process more efficient. Tele–home care can link into primary care consultation systems, enabling primary care physician, patient, and nurse to teleconsult. Fears of tele–home care reducing the need for community nurses are probably unfounded. With the need for home care services rising and a limited supply of nurses, tele–home care is a way of enabling community nurses to work more efficiently and keep pace with the demand[177] for their services. A feasibility study of telehealth in home hospice care showed that patients were satisfied with telehealth and found it easy to use the equipment.[178] It also helped them to become more active partners in their own health care.

For patients, tele–home care offers the prospect of establishing tele–home care communities. These allow homebound patients to make contact with similar patients through videoconferencing, a "virtual ward" analogous to the hospital ward except in the community. These areas of health care are evolving rapidly. They promise to bring enormous changes in how patients and community nurses interact. More data are needed to understand how patients and nurses feel about these changes so that the process of care can be driven by factors other than just cost.

Establishing Evidence That Tele–Home Care Services Will Save Costs, Improve Quality, or Increase Market Share for the Health Care Organization Being Approached to Buy Telehealth Services

Tele–home care can increase the efficiency of on-site home nursing by reducing the time spent driving.[179] It can halve the cost of a home visit with no detriment to quality or participant satisfaction, and it allows a home nurse to care for 15 to 22 patients per day compared to 5 per day using conventional home visiting. A feasibility study of hospice care suggests that there are 33%–50% savings on the cost of nursing visits for palliative care at home if tele–home care is used in place of conventional home visits.[178]

Establish a Market for Home Care Telehealth Services If These Are Offered

The number of elderly people in the population is rising. Health care practice is changing, and the costs of telehealth technologies are falling. The use of telehealth in home care is likely to rise dramatically. Although high-technology applications in telehealth, such as remote surgery, are great technical accomplishments, they are typically high-cost, low-volume applications for telehealth. The real growth potential for telehealth is in consumer-led, high-volume, low-cost health care applications. Tele–home care may become one of the quintessential telehealth applications on which the rapid growth of remote care will be based.

A range of projects, including hospital-at-home schemes (in the United Kingdom), stroke care at home, palliative care, and AIDS care in the community all lend themselves to the addition of this new technology. In the United Kingdom the home nursing visit is currently an inefficient way to manage patients at home. The community nurse usually drives to see the patient to make an assessment. Specialist care or treatment, if required, may take another visit. An initial remote tele-home consultation can establish whether the patient should be seen by a specialist and avoid an unnecessary visit or can prepare any special treatment required and take it directly to the patient.

An expensive problem in community-based health care in many countries, including the United Kingdom and the United States, is at the interface between home care for nursing and home care for social reasons. The use of telehealth increases the potential for using generic workers who have health care and social care skills to care for people at home and save costs. If a generic care worker has a particular concern for a client's health she/he can use tele–home care to conduct joint video assessments with community nurses. If the client needs a visit from a nurse or a specific treatment, such as for a pressure sore, this can be arranged more quickly than with the conventional delivery of services. Making interagency services such as this requires training, agreed-on care protocols, arrangements for joint management of the service and, most crucially, budgetary flexibility.

Remote monitoring of patients at home is another major growth market for telehealth. An established commercial market already exists, with people paying for their own home monitoring to detect cardiac dysfunction. The technology for remote monitoring of physiological function is developing most rapidly in the area of sports medicine. Athletes can buy inexpensive monitoring devices to access physiological parameters like pulse and blood pressure while they exercise. The adaptation of these mass-produced devices is likely to provide the future technology for home monitoring in health care. Custom technologies adapted from hospital monitoring devices are usually prohibitively expensive to use in home monitoring situations. The growth of the home monitoring market for the care of acute illness at home awaits the linkage of inexpensive monitoring devices to expert systems that can assess predictive patterns of abnormal physiological events.

The limiting factor to widespread home monitoring of patients is likely to be creating intelligent systems to interpret the data from home monitoring and recognize abnormal physiological events. Our anecdotal experience of monitoring patients with respiratory disease at home shows it is difficult to define safe normative values to use when monitoring physiological variables in the home environment. The variation in physiological readings at home can be greater than the normal values defined in hospital settings. If the narrower range of normal values developed in hospital settings is used inappropriately for home monitoring, false alarms can result. Such false alarms are important because the cost of assessing patients at home and inappropriate hospital admissions can make home monitoring more expensive than conventional care. Intelligent systems to interpret the readout from monitors, now under development, can detect patterns of readings and interactions among multiple physiological variables and so detect true abnormalities earlier.

Ensuring That a Telehealth Home Care Program Sells Its Product and Not the General Idea of Buying Telehealth

The tele–home care market forms part of the overall market for primary care services. As we mentioned previously, the complexity of this market is about developing people networks around the care of the patient rather than specific technical considerations.

There is a primary market for the sale of the telehealth equipment and a secondary market for the delivery of telehealth services in tele–home care as in other areas of telehealth. The product involved in delivering home health care services using telehealth is complex. It is an organizational model of care delivery to people at home, not merely supplying the equipment. If a telehealth program approaches a prospective client with the equipment and well-thought-through models of care delivery, the client is unlikely to want to look elsewhere in the current market for tele–home care.

INTERNATIONAL TELEHEALTH MARKETS, INCLUDING TRAVEL REPATRIATION

A large and growing international market for telehealth is impossible to quantitate because there are no accurate data available. Countries such as the United States and the United Kingdom have the capacity to export health care expertise to less developed countries; early examples were the Middle East,[180] China, and other parts of Asia. Assessing the commercial success of these ventures is difficult to gauge. The initial promise seems in many cases to be more than the ultimate financial reward. The costs of the technology and data transmission are very high. The paucity of financial data reported and dearth of commercial companies starting up to provide international health care services is probably the best evidence that this is currently a market opportunity rather than a commercial success story in telehealth.

The market for health care services using telehealth is not robust enough nor have needs assessments been done to accurately predict what this market will be. We usually caution academic medical centers against an unfettered entrepreneurial spirit in establishing high-cost commercial telehealth links to other countries before they have made a commercial success of local and regional networks. We do not have the data to advise whether a survival strategy for large academic medical centers is to export their current expertise to less developed countries. In the longer term they may be doing these countries a disservice and only temporarily delaying their own need to restructure how they deliver care themselves.

In contrast to the supply of medical expertise using telehealth, the supply of telehealth equipment to enable the development of local and regional networks within countries is a commercial success story. Commercial telehealth opportunities are developing in the medical repatriation of vacationers and people working abroad to their home countries. Health insurers who cover holiday travel have major concerns about the cost and appropriateness of care received by people when traveling abroad. We know of many anecdotal instances where overseas clinics have run up large and unnecessary medical bills in managing patients. For medicolegal reasons travel insurance companies often felt powerless to refuse to pay such bills in acute medical emergencies. Many travel health insurers have developed networks of physicians and hospital providers abroad whom they trust to institute care only when appropriate. As these networks are developing, the case for telemedicine is also growing, although the business case for implementation is still lagging behind.

RURAL HEALTH CARE MARKETS

Rural health care is an area where much of the future growth of telehealth has been predicated. There is a very good case to suggest that there will be a big market for telehealth in rural areas because of the distances from health care services and the time it takes to reach them. In the United States the Federal Communications Commission established a Universal Services Fund in January 1998. This program subsidizes the costs of providing digital data services in rural areas, trying to align them with prices in urban areas. The program presupposes that the cost of bandwidth is a major limiting factor to telehealth expansion in rural areas. Although telehealth use has expanded rapidly in the United States in response to federal grants,[22] this has not always been matched by a corresponding buildup of the consultation rates necessary to sustain such programs in the long term.

The long-term commercial success of rural telehealth networks ultimately depends on developing the revenue to support them. In rural areas the low geographical density of physicians and nurses means telehealth cannot totally substitute for conventional health care delivery systems. Cost savings in rural areas are difficult to realize because of the need to maintain arrangements for face-to-face consultations and emergency transport systems remain regardless of telehealth. The reorganization of health care services needed to deliver the savings to pay for commercial telehealth services is difficult to achieve. Also, in the United States the future of commercial telehealth services to rural areas may be linked to the growth of managed care.[181] This has been a disappointing area of growth despite the 1997 Balanced Budget Act.

If the provision of telehealth to rural areas does not make commercial sense and digital data service subsidies do not make a difference, then the market for telehealth in rural areas may have to be determined by social policy decisions. In the United Kingdom universal health care provision includes equity as a criteria for providing services, so the rural/urban disparity is less obvious than in the United States. In the United Kingdom, inequalities in health care due to geographical distance and low populations are determined by national formulas for the distribution of health care resources. Taxpayers in urban areas may subsidize rural health care indirectly through taxation. Whether this same subsidy will be needed for telehealth is unclear. Neither the health care market nor government social policy statements have made a clear decision about telehealth.

THE MILITARY AND THE MARKET
FOR TELEHEALTH

No discussion of telehealth would be complete without mentioning the contribution of the military to telehealth. Many of the dramatic applications for telehealth have been developed by the US military for use in conflict situations such as the Gulf War,[13] Bosnia,[182] and other arenas. The US military has taken a strategic view of telehealth in keeping with the global scope of their operations.[183] They have explored technical aspects of virtual presence that may transform our concepts of what telehealth can do in the future.[184] The role of the US military is changing, and since the end of the cold war its technology, including telehealth, is becoming available to commercial applications. The US military has had and will continue to have a significant role in determining the frontiers in the market for telehealth technology. Its focus of interest is currently switching to low-cost high-volume applications. An example of a military-linked collaboration is an initiative called "Good Medicine in Bad Places," a Web-based information exchange using low-cost technology.

MARKETS FOR TELEHEALTH: A SUMMARY

It is difficult to predict the future market for telehealth because of the volatility of events. In early 1998 the instability in the Asian financial markets had repercussions for the export of telehealth equipment to Asia. In the same way, health care markets are volatile in the United Kingdom and the United States. Some major health care providers are in deep financial trouble, making these health care markets uncertain for telehealth equipment and service providers. In this volatility we believe there are considerable opportunities for telehealth to solve otherwise insoluble problems in delivering health care services. A market for telehealth exists where there are opportunities to sell equipment and services.

We expect to see a growing expansion in the market for telehealth equipment that will precede any major growth in the market for health care services using telehealth. We believe that the market for telehealth is like the early market for the telephone and the facsimile machine. When a health care provider is one of a few with the technology of telehealth, there are limited ways for the provider to use the technology to change the process of care. The real expansion in telemedicine depends on networks of telehealth users reaching critical mass, thus allowing the organizational changes that telehealth can bring to happen. This growth will happen suddenly. The telehealth market may be governed by complexity, not linear dynamics. If so, telehealth companies may experience increasing and disproportionately large returns to scale on investment. The real challenge facing markets for telehealth is how to transform point-to-point telemedicine applications into larger national/international networks—networks where the capacity to transfer surplus capacity and reduce health care costs can be realized.

8

Contracting for Telehealth Services

THE IMPORTANCE OF CONTRACTING
TO TELEHEALTH SERVICES

Ninety percent of telehealth programs are currently grant-funded, and most of these either do not or cannot sustain themselves commercially in the market-driven health care environments in which they have to operate. As long as market-driven health care systems prevail as the way in which health care is delivered, contracting for telehealth is a crucial issue. Often the directors of telehealth programs view the benefits of telehealth in general and of their telehealth program in particular as self-evident. They expect financial support for the program to be forthcoming when the grant support ends. Telehealth is in its third incarnation over a period of 20 years. It is unlikely that telehealth programs as we see them in our current health care environment will survive unless they show creativity and entrepreneurship in attracting resources. We believe creative contracting as much as technological advance will decide the future shape of telehealth over the next seven years and whether formal interest in telehealth will be sustained. Although the decreasing cost of equipment means telehealth will inevitably happen, the default position will be the same chaos as the use of the telephone.

In many instances where telehealth services are introduced they cut across the traditional ways of delivering health care services. That they do so is one of their strengths, but it is also their weakness. They do not readily fit into existing contracting systems from which the revenue they need to survive can be derived. A lot of energy is being expended to try to secure government support for telehealth reimbursement by public health systems in the United Kingdom, the United States, and Canada. Telehealth companies must look for new, creative ways to contract for health care services if they are going to prosper and grow. Governments are currently prepared to fund health care innovation such as telehealth on two conditions:

1. If they feel the market will sustain the health care innovation once the government "pump priming" ends.
2. If the health care innovation can provide evidence-based, cost-effective health care services to sections of society where government has identified a need and the market is either unable or unwilling to meet this need.
3. If a targeted group lobbies for its use.

In this chapter we look at possible sources of contract revenue for telehealth companies and how payers in health care are searching for providers who can give evidence of the clinical effectiveness, population need, and cost-effectiveness of their services. We believe the long-term future of telehealth will be in pursuing contracts based on outcomes, not fee-for-service contracts.

THE TELEHEALTH AND GOVERNMENT REIMBURSEMENT DEBATE: NATIONAL AND LOCAL PERSPECTIVES

The government funds public health care services in the United Kingdom through supporting the National Health Service (NHS). The US government offers elements of publicly funded health care through Medicare, and the states provide health care through Medicaid, using both state and federal dollars. When health care innovators tried to change the way health care services were delivered in the past, they often relied on the government to pay. This reliance on government has taken place in the United Kingdom because of the way government, through the NHS, is responsible for delivering the vast majority of health care services. In the United States, 50% of care is delivered privately; however, whatever lead the Health Care Financing Administration (HCFA) takes on health care reimbursement issues the private insurance sector often follows.

Since 1991 health care delivery in the United Kingdom by the NHS has taken place in a market environment with purchasers and providers of care. Although a central executive takes overall responsibility for the NHS, the day-to-day purchasing of health care services has now been devolved down to local purchasing authorities linked to primary care practitioners. Each year purchasers of health care in the NHS have continued to receive revenue increases to cover inflation. However, since 1995 many local purchasers of health care have been asked to make cash-releasing savings of between 3% and 6% on the revenue they receive each year to provide services to their local population. These savings have been made from either reducing the direct provision of health care services, reducing the administrative costs of delivering care, or running up a deficit. Although there is an argument to suggest that tough financial circumstances may encourage health care innovation because health care providers will adopt technologies such as telehealth to make them more efficient, this has not been the general experience in the United Kingdom for various reasons. The effect of recent health care changes in the United Kingdom is that the government is now less prepared to sponsor a new health care innovation such as telehealth unless it is clearly based on evidence that it is both effective and cost-effective. In the absence of this evidence to clearly support telehealth, neither the UK government nor the NHS has a definitive policy on telehealth. Both clearly show interest in telehealth and recognize its potential for delivering health care services more efficiently and effectively in the future.

In the United States HCFA established a series of telemedicine projects in 1996 to look at the implications of the remote delivery of health care on the contracting and financing of health care services. The particular concern in the United States about these projects was to look at the cost implications for Medicare of reimbursing for telemedicine. Telemedicine has a potential to reduce the costs of health care delivery and make it more efficient. It also has the potential to add considerably to cost inflation in health care. The federal government in the United States has encouraged telemedicine development through making grants available, particularly to the military. For obvious reasons it did not want to provide a blank check to fund the unevaluated uptake of telehealth into the general health care environment. At a state level, where the funding of Medicaid is administered, there has been much more interest in funding telehealth projects. The product champions for telehealth at the individual state level in the United States are often individual state governors. Governors with an interest in telehealth are not united by their political persuasion as Democrats or Republicans but by their common vision that information technology can change the delivery of services to their citizens. The Western Governors' Association is an influential group with a published vision of telehealth as part of a broader reconfiguration of government services through information technology that includes

+ Schools and libraries
+ Access to government departments
+ Prison care
+ Further education
+ Representative government

The reason for mentioning this change of government attitude in the United Kingdom and United States for the reimbursement of telehealth service is to dispel any notion that governments will uncritically fund telehealth because it is a "good thing." This is naive in the extreme. The basis of contracting in telehealth cannot be of telehealth programs presenting a fait accompli of "take it or leave it" and presenting a bill. Telehealth programs must understand for which telehealth services government agencies are willing to reimburse and demonstrate that they can provide these effectively and at a competitive cost. The HCFA Medicare Telemedicine Demonstration in the United States is a good illustration of the important issues that health care purchasers in the public and private sector have voiced about contracting for telehealth in both the United Kingdom and the United States.

THE HCFA TELEMEDICINE DEMONSTRATION PROJECT AS AN INDICATION OF THE CONTRACTING ISSUES IN THE PURCHASING OF TELEHEALTH SERVICES

The HCFA project started on October 1, 1996, with the specific task of looking at reimbursement for telehealth services. It runs until September 30, 1999, and its working "rules" are as follows:

+ Reimbursement will apply only to situations where live teleconsultations are undertaken.
+ Reimbursement for telemedicine services apply to only a set number of treatment codes that cover outpatient evaluation and management at the spoke, office consultation at the hub, and evaluation and management of inpatients and inpatient consultation.
+ When eligible telehealth reimbursement conditions are met, the consultant at the hub gets his/her full fee paid, and the referring primary care physician gets 50% of his/her fee as reimbursement for his/her work component.
+ The health care provider can get up to 100% reimbursement for the cost of providing the telehealth facility.
+ At certain selected sites there is a 20% reduction in practitioner

reimbursement if the patient is admitted to hospital for an inpatient stay as a result of the teleconsultation.
+ The project intends to look at a single "bundled payment" for the service.

The HCFA research study expects to collect data from 600 teleconsultations and 2,500 conventional consultations and will analyze the clinical behavior and the costs.

Financial concerns prompted the HCFA health study. They and other health care purchasers are alarmed at the prospect that they will inadvertently create the wrong financial incentives to stimulate the growth of telehealth. Health care purchasers do not want to see the rapid adoption of new technologies such as videoconsultation by health care providers without ensuring that there are simultaneous benefits from either reductions in the cost or increase in the quality of care. These fears are illustrated by how reimbursement for videoconsultation could interplay with use of the telephone, an existing telehealth system that is in widespread use already.

In chapter 1 we discussed how telephone consultation is now a ubiquitous and vital part of routine health care delivery in the United Kingdom and United States. Health care purchasers often do not directly pay for the costs of telephone consultation as items of service in charges for the health care services they buy. These costs are absorbed within the current contractual systems that pay for the general delivery of services. If HCFA or any other health care purchaser directly reimburses health care providers for teleconsultations, then what may happen is that current health care activity that takes place on the telephone may switch to become a videoconsultation. Unless this change from telephone to videoconsultation results in more efficient management of patients, the net effect will be inflation in health care costs. The implications for health care purchasers and insurers of getting telehealth reimbursement wrong are the reasons they are moving cautiously on this issue. Many telehealth programs look at the HCFA project as a possible stalking horse for the eventual arrival of fee-for-service telehealth reimbursement. There is an obvious "pot of gold at the end of the rainbow" argument supporting a push for fee-for-service reimbursement as a revenue source for telehealth programs. This is an improbable future scenario for how health care purchasing organizations will contract for telehealth services. We believe this is improbable for three main reasons.

1.   We only see fee-for-service as a deliberate tool of government policy to attract health care services into underserved areas. That HCFA has agreed to reimbursement for telehealth services in rural areas in their first general

telehealth demonstration projects is a reflection of this policy. Lack of adequate health care is one of the factors that make rural areas unpopular to live in and contribute to rural depopulation. It does not therefore follow that there will be general reimbursement for telehealth everywhere on a fee-for-service basis just because of rural health care needs.

2.   The additional costs of billing for telehealth as individual fee-for-service items will raise the administrative costs of delivering health care. It will also raise the potential for fraud.

3.   The general trend in contracting by health care systems is moving away from fee-for-service contracts and toward capitation-based systems that underwrite health for a defined population.

FEE-FOR-SERVICE CONTRACTS AND TELEHEALTH

Fee-for-service payment contracts mean that health care providers, whether practitioners or organizations, receive a previously agreed-on fee for each item of service they deliver. Examples of the different kinds of items of service included in a fee-for-service contract are gallbladder operations performed by a surgeon and home visits undertaken by a community nurse. Fee-for-service was one of the reasons for the rapid inflation in health care costs in the United States in the 1970s, 1980s, and early 1990s.

Many telehealth programs see fee-for-service as the ideal way to contract for telehealth services and get the revenue they need to survive. These programs envisage the contracting process as simply billing a hospital, health care purchaser, or health care insurer for each telehealth consultation. This strategy may not work for one major practical and one major strategic reason. The practical reason is that the volume of telehealth consultations performed by most telehealth programs is low. Low-volume consultation makes it difficult to cover the costs of a telehealth program from revenues generated by fees paid for items of service. With low volumes, the costs per consultation will be much higher than purchasers will pay. A variant of the fee-for-service contracting method is for telehealth to offer a cost and volume contract, where a telehealth program contracts to supply up to a predetermined level of teleconsultations at a set price. Again, the problem is what to do if the volumes of consultations don't occur.

The strategic reason that fee-for-service may not work for telehealth programs as a contracting system in the future is that health care purchasers are trying to move away from fee-for-service and cost and volume contracting. They are looking for other ways to contract, and telehealth programs will have more success with health care purchasers if they look for more creative solutions to cement the relationships they are trying to form.

In the United Kingdom, fee-for-service contracts were once widely used by the NHS to encourage behavioral change in practitioners, such as encouraging general practitioners to increase the rate of cervical smears and dentists to treat patients. Fee-for-service is still widely used by private medicine in the United States and United Kingdom to reimburse practitioners and organizations for the procedures they perform. A legacy of the previous fee-for-service culture prevailing in health care is the contracting information collected by the public sectors of the health care systems in the United Kingdom and the United States. Typically, this contracting information records the activities of the professionals working in a service, not the outcomes for the patients treated by the interventions of these health care professionals.

Health care purchasers no longer blindly accept that a health care intervention will necessarily result in improved health for patients. Increasingly, they are looking for contracts based on measures of improvement in the health of patients, not just the activities performed by the health care professionals. They see fee-for-service contracts as a simplistic way of purchasing health care service, a way that rewards health care providers for performing procedures without ensuring that they improve the health of the patients they see. The goal is increasingly for health care contracting in publicly funded health care services to reflect the outcome of treatment for diseases; for example, diabetes and hypertension. The focus of health care contracting is moving away from buying simple processes of care toward buying packages of care associated with measurable health outcomes for patients. These outcomes must demonstrate how disease is treated and whether symptoms are relieved. Other trends in health care purchasing and providing that discourage fee-for-service contracting are the increasing movement to managed care and capitated funding of health care services.

Health care contracting is becoming more sophisticated, reflecting the complexity of the process of delivering health care now. Health care purchasers fit broadly into two types. In the first category the health purchaser purchases public health care, managed care, and capitated care. These purchasers would like to contract more strategically with health care providers and use contracts based on prices for improving the health of populations. They would like to leave the fine details of the process of care to providers. The second category of health purchaser, typically a health care insurer, continues to deal with processes of care and favors fee-for-service contracts. They see their situation changing with the inroads of managed care into their markets and with government legislation of health insurance. Legislation such as the Health Insurance Portability and Accountability Act of 1996

(HIPAA) in the United States encourages insurers to take a more population-based approach and to discriminate less against individuals.

These changes in health care purchasing give messages to telehealth programs that are struggling with how to become commercially viable, messages saying they must view telehealth in a wider context than just reimbursement for telehealth transactions. We see fee-for-service contracting in telehealth persisting only within the framework of larger processes of care. Our belief in this stems from the growth that we are seeing in teleradiology in the United States. HCFA is not sure how many teleradiology consultations it now pays for per year because it pays for radiology services and leaves it to the provider to decide exactly how the processes of x-ray reporting and film storage take place. Some teleradiology service providers contract to provide teleradiology services on a fee-for-service basis to other health care organizations, who in turn contract with health care purchasers. This works because the teleradiology provider is entrepreneurial and is able to offer value-added services to another health care provider that make the service more competitive than using conventional radiology services.

Contracting directly with health care purchasers in new and more complex ways takes time to develop. We do not see the advantage in passively waiting for reimbursement systems to evolve. In the short term we see considerably more scope for telehealth service providers developing fee-for-service and cost and volume contracts through subcontracting their services to other health care providers. A major future role for serious commercial telehealth programs is to "facilities manage" the processes of providing remote health care services to hospitals, hospital groups, and health maintenance organizations.

As a facilities management service the responsibility of the telehealth program is less about the overall process of care or the health of the patient. The direct management of this element of service is the responsibility of the health care provider with whom they are subcontracting. The responsibility of the telehealth service provider is thereby limited to facilitating remote health care transactions efficiently to set specifications. These specifications have to be set through close collaborative work with the health care provider to identify exactly where telehealth can add value or can save costs for their service. Reimbursement for these services on a fee-for-service basis then makes sense. The concept of telehealth service providers as facilities management services means that the future growth of telehealth services may depend on managing complex collaborative arrangements between health care providers and telecommunications companies. We will explore the contracting implications of this later in this chapter and the business and management implications in later chapters.

CONTRACTING FOR TELEHEALTH SERVICES IN CAPITATED CARE AND MANAGED CARE SITUATIONS

Capitated care and managed care systems are similar. They provide a set level of funding to cover the health needs of a specified population. Examples of capitated care are the purchase of general health care by health authorities in the United Kingdom and the provision of some Medicare-funded services under capitated care arrangements with the HCFA in the United States. Managed care accounts for increasing proportions of health care in the United States. One long-term scenario resulting from the 1991 health care reforms in the United Kingdom is that they may create a similar managed care arrangement to that gradually evolving in the United States.

Capitated care and managed care offer receptive environments for developing a whole range of telehealth services from primary prevention to palliative care. To understand where these opportunities exist for telehealth in managed and capitated care means appreciating the very different approaches these systems take to delivering health care services. Commercial success under fee-for-service reimbursement usually makes maximizing revenue equate crudely to delivering the maximum amount of services as often as possible. In contrast to this, delivering health care services under managed and capitated care funding makes the main commercial incentive to provide the minimum quantity of care appropriate for the population and do this as efficiently as possible. The success formulas for these two systems are shown in Figure 8.1.

Failure to appreciate this cultural difference among types of organization may make it very difficult for telehealth service providers when they negotiate contracts to provide services for managed care organizations. The underlying contracting strategy of most telehealth providers is solely driven by the cost dynamics of providing remote health care. This dynamic is based on a

Fee for service

Commercial success = providing as many services as can be sold

8.1a

Capitated Care and Managed Care

Commercial success = providing care as efficiently as possible and at the volume that is most appropriate to improving the health of the population

8.1b

Figure 8.1   Commercial success under different reinbursement systems.

premise that they must maximize the volume of services they sell to lower their operating costs, boost demand, and therefore generate profits. They are following classical economic theory in trying to make demand for their services equate to what they supply at the "right" price. Capitated care and managed care organizations may not be looking at telehealth as a simple product to provide to the populations they serve. Less obvious reasons for why managed care organizations are interested in contracting for service such as telehealth are given in Table 8.1.

Telehealth has yet to capture the public imagination to the extent that people are willing to pay more to receive it or to trade other opportunities for care they currently receive for it. Where capitated care and managed care organizations are eager to explore contracting for telehealth is where it reduces their costs or complements areas they are developing in their own services at no additional cost.

Contracting successfully to provide services to capitated care and managed care organizations often requires a more sophisticated approach to negotiating than just selling a projected volume of fee-for-service cases. Developing a positive case for introducing telehealth services into a managed care organization usually requires taking a wider perspective of the health care situations they manage. This type of approach is illustrated by the example of taking a managed care organization through different scenarios for adopting telehealth to remotely manage trauma care cases. Tables 8.2 and 8.3 help to develop a business case for remote trauma care by progressively moving away from purely cost per case considerations.

CONTRACTING TO PROVIDE TELEHEALTH IN EMERGENCY CARE

The case for contracting to provide telehealth support to a remote emergency room in a rural area from a major trauma center for a capitated care or managed care organization may show the cost projections in Table 8.2 when viewed in purely fee-for-service terms.

If the equivalent cost of conventionally managing these trauma cases is $45 per consultation, it is difficult to make the case for partially replacing the conventional mode of service delivery with a telehealth system. At first glance it seems that there is no economic case for contracting to provide telehealth for remote trauma management with this health maintenance organization.

Contract negotiations might finish there, but an advantage of working in managed care environments is the incentive to work with protocols for

Table 8.1   Reasons for Managed Care Systems Contracting for Telehealth

1. It will attract a larger capitated population or more members. An economic caveat to this is that they must not then have to pay out more in providing the telehealth service than they can expect to receive in income from any new capitated population/membership it brings in.
2. It will reduce the costs and/or improve the quality of the service they offer at no extra cost.
3. It fits with an area of service development they are pursuing at no cost or negligible marginal cost.
4. They feel obliged to offer the service because in a competitive environment they feel they will lose membership to other managed care organizations if they do not.

care and to look at data on patient outcomes. Using outcome data from protocol-driven care and incorporating telehealth may give the case for a telehealth contract a new and different complexion, as shown in Table 8.3. An analysis of these data shows a positive effect from using videoconsultation. It has substantially altered the clinical care of individual patients in 24 of the 70 cases. These changes in clinical care for 24 cases can then be examined further to see if they translate into cost savings, as shown in Table 8.4.

It does not automatically follow from an analysis of remote trauma such as this that a telehealth system is necessarily the only or even most appropriate solution. Some of the savings projected for telehealth could also result from changes to existing protocols and clinical training using conventional care. The example shows how making the case for using telehealth often means being prepared to look at the process of delivering health care and not just making a superficial analysis of patient utilization data.

A new area where telehealth service providers are contracting with managed care organizations is in providing Internet-based services to patients, particularly health information services. Many managed care organizations have their own Web sites to communicate directly with patients. Once they have established this facility for themselves, the marginal cost for a managed care organization of linking their Web site to other telehealth services or

Table 8.2   Costs per Consultation of Providing Remote Trauma Consultation

Projected no. of trauma referrals for videoconsultation per year	70
Consultation costs for videoconsultation referrals per year	$7,000
Overhead costs of providing videoconsultation per year	$28,000
Costs per consultation	$500

Table 8.3   Changes in Care Protocols Resulting from Videoconsultation

Changes to care management resulting in improved outcomes for orthopedic cases as a result of referral for videoconsultation	9
Number of cases in which the management of head-injured patients would change after referral for videoconsultation	12
Projected number of cases in which the risk of litigation would be saved by videoconsultation	3

buying additional content to repackage for their own Web site is low. Contracting to offer Internet-based health services to HMOs can be complicated because of ensuring the security of patient data. Existing telehealth service providers are often rigid about definitions and feel that videoconferencing using ISDN and asynchronous training mode (ATM) is synonymous with telehealth. All future scenarios for telehealth must include using the Internet as a possible option. Providing a service, not a preoccupation with the medium used, is what will be important to achieving commercial success in telehealth.

In summary, we believe there is major growth potential for telehealth services in working closely with capitated care and managed care organizations to offer telehealth as a way of delivering substantial cost savings. Cost savings in these situations usually result from using telehealth to alter traditional ways of providing care. Growing opportunities exist to offer managed care organizations a wide range of telehealth services, from disease prevention to direct treatment on a wide range of media, including the Internet. These activities are areas where telehealth providers have a role in working with pharmaceutical companies and capitated care/managed care organizations to formalize telehealth into the disease management program being developed. Telehealth then becomes an integral part of protocols for delivering effective care.

Table 8.4   Costs Savings Associated with Videoconsultation

Cost savings of altered management of fractures from earlier surgery, reductions in hospital stay and aftercare	$12,600
Cost savings from reductions in the transport costs of head-injured patients and the more efficient management of multiple–trauma patients	$25,000
Reduced risk in litigation from the recognition of subarachnoid hemorrhage, opiate overdose, and thoracic aneurysm	? many $0000s
Cost saving in patient management from videoconsultation	$37,600+

CONTRACTING FOR DISEASE MANAGEMENT

The majority of health care now provided in developed countries is focused on treating chronic diseases—diseases affecting people over a long period of time and for which there are usually no curative treatments. People with these conditions are cared for in a multiplicity of settings at various stages of their disease and receive a wide variety of different treatments. Established ways of delivering treatment are usually geared to dealing reactively with symptoms if and when they occur. Rarely does the care fit within formal long-term strategies for the management of the chronic disease process itself. Health care purchasers now want contracts for the services they buy to bring together what seem chaotic regimens to manage individuals with chronic diseases into coherent treatment protocols. Treatment protocols include features like those described in Table 8.5.

People differ in their individual susceptibility to disease. Diseases themselves can also vary in their severity and the manifestation of the effects they produce. The main skill needed to devise workable disease management protocols is in making them applicable to the broad range of people of different sex, ethnicity, age group, educational background, and emotional response who present to clinicians in day-to-day clinical practice. A good protocol for the care of this range of people with chronic diseases may work in managing only 65%–90% of cases seen in routine clinical care. Any protocol seeking to manage 100% of cases usually becomes so complex as to be unworkable. This often makes the main practical problem with using protocol-driven care one of deciding how to manage the exceptional cases (10%–35%) not fitting into the protocol. People often don't fit into the criteria of a protocol because of their own idiosyncrasies or those of the disease process. One approach to this problem is to staff the service with practitioners who are trained to deal with the exceptional 10%–35% of cases and who are then overqualified to manage the other 65%–95% of cases. This solution raises the service costs, and there is a risk of practitioners becoming bored and complacent when they are overqualified to deal with routine cases fitting within the protocol.

A second solution is to refine the protocol even more, to the extent that it covers all eventualities. This refinement is usually a practical impossibility. It may mean repeatedly revising the protocols and then training clinical staff in updated versions at considerable expense. A third possibility is to use telehealth. Protocols can be kept broad and simple and use staff appropriately qualified to work within the protocol. Telehealth comes into play to offer specialist expertise in the exceptional cases where disease management protocols do not apply. This third solution is even more effective when the

Table 8.5   Essentials of Treatment Protocols for Disease Management

1. They are based on evidence of clinical effectiveness and include prevention, screening, diagnosis, treatment, and palliation where appropriate.
2. They consider the most appropriate setting for the patient to receive care, e.g., home, clinic, hospital, hospice.
3. They include information for patients about treatment options and the risks and benefits of treatment.
4. They include a formal clinical audit process and measurement tools to provide information on outcomes.
5. They are consistent, and they assign responsibility for the delivery of care and providing information to patients unambiguously and without unnecessary duplication.

specialist consultation service link is arranged with the clinicians responsible for devising the protocol. Protocol development for disease management and this model of remote consultation service are revenue opportunities for specialist academic medical centers. The advantages of using telehealth in disease management protocols are shown in Table 8.6.

A disease management approach in contracting to deliver services is in its infancy and inevitably makes the work of incorporating telehealth more complicated. The telehealth contractor may be asked to act as more than a facilities management service and more as a health care provider in the way described in the previous remote trauma care example in managed care (Tables 8.2–8.4). Disease management takes a telehealth service into the realms of directly delivering health care services and actively managing the clinical care of patients remotely. The telehealth provider may then face the prospect of employing clinicians directly or under a subcontracting arrangement. Employing clinicians creates greater complexity for the operation of the telehealth program, particularly in relation to the clinical interface with other services. Is the telehealth organization then a health care provider offering telehealth? Complexities such as these have already arisen in trying to devise contracting frameworks to enable prison health care systems to use telehealth. Examining some of the issues raised in contracting for prison care illustrates the range of challenges a telehealth program faces when it is asked to deliver health care services directly.

CONTRACTING TO PROVIDE PRISON HEALTH CARE USING TELEHEALTH

Delivering any health care service usually involves a complex series of interrelated processes, and frequently the operational details are ill-defined. Lack

Table 8.6   Advantages of Telehealth in Disease Management Protocols

- Consistency in the application of the protocol
- Including more patients in the protocol
- Direct feedback into future refinement of the protocol
- Reduced clinical risk
- Increased patient confidence
- Direct education and training for the staff using the protocols
- Immediate warnings of any adverse reactions or contraindications

of clear operational roles and responsibilities creates problems when contracting to provide telehealth services. Prison health care arrangements are usually well demarcated because of security considerations. In the United States a rising prison population and concerns about its impact on the quality and cost of health care provision has prompted many states to change the way they deliver prison health care and to include telehealth services within their system. The prime motivation of states for considering telehealth are saving costs and improving the quality of care, and it helps in introducing this to have the health care service requirements well demarcated.

Prison systems usually have to meet the direct costs of providing health care and also pay to guard and transport prisoners to hospitals when outside medical expertise is required, often paying overtime rates to do so. These combined expenses may then come from the overall budget for custodial services for the whole prison population. Telehealth can reduce the requirement to transport prisoners to outside health care facilities for medical advice and offer the possibility of considerable cost savings. Prison health care is effectively a capitated care system, and states are trying to make cost savings by tactically contracting out health delivery to organizations offering telehealth in their service portfolio. This contracting out is justifiable only if the telehealth service provider is able to deliver a service of at least comparable quality as the one it is replacing and at reduced cost. When a telehealth provider bids for these contracts, it must have expertise in the operational management of health care services and project management of a sizable information technology installation.

The dual complexity of information technology and health care provision makes a consortium arrangement for providing services an attractive arrangement in prison telehealth. Telehealth service providers can therefore find themselves having to take the lead role in bringing together a consortium whose remit is to offer capitated health care arrangements to provide health care to a prison population. When this happens, the key elements to success are clear and binding contractual arrangements among the parties involved in the consortium that blend with tight, jointly agreed service specifications with the state prison system. These key elements can be neglected, particularly when grant-funded telehealth programs are attracted to providing prison medicine as a safe first foothold in an unfamiliar commercial world. There should be at least 14 key criteria that must be covered by both sides in this contracting process, as shown in Table 8.7.

A frequent mistake made by health care organizations in general and by telehealth programs in particular is to pursue new business and regard the actual contract as an afterthought, just a loose end to tie up. As it makes the decision to go for a contract, a telehealth organization must begin framing the operational specification of the service and judge whether there is a sufficient margin in delivering this service specification to justify their bidding. It is often a disaster when this process starts in earnest only after the contract has been awarded. This is how budgets overrun, services fail to deliver, and reputations are destroyed.

THE CONTRACTING PROCESS

The difference between being an aspiring telehealth service provider and a commercial success is measured in terms of having agreed-on contracts to provide services and being able to deliver these services. In the changing health care environments of the United States and United Kingdom contracting arrangements to provide commercial telehealth services can include those in the list shown in Table 8.8.

Table 8.7   Minimum Contract Criteria in Contracting for Telehealth

1. Exact clinical and technical specifications for the service
2. Financial viability linked to clear payment mechanisms
3. Clarification on competitive pricing arrangements and contract duration
4. Explicit outline of how to deliver the clinical service efficiently and effectively
5. The capacity to deliver remote consultations to specification
6. Adequate premises and clinic space
7. Prearranged interface with other health care providers and billing arrangements
8. All regulatory requirements outlined and met
9. Clinical and financial risk management systems described
10. Quality standards agreed on and arrangements to monitor them outlined
11. Clear legal associations and indemnity arrangements
12. Contract monitoring and information requirements formalized
13. Emergency arrangements in place for the unexpected or disaster situations
14. Payment and conciliation processes in case of disagreements

Table 8.8   Common Contractual Arrangements for Commercial Telehealth

1. Fee-for-service/cost and volume contracts
2. Subcontracts with another health care provider
3. Lead provider in a consortium, e.g., prison health service contract
4. Outcomes-based capitated care contracts.

Because telehealth programs can be relatively new organizations, or start-ups, contract income is usually the most important issue for a telehealth service provider. These four different contracting methods each provides a different level of financial reward and different incentives for a telehealth provider. We place no value judgment on which method is used. We recommend that, if possible, different options be explored because each can make a big difference to the level of return. The precision with which the contract to deliver telehealth services is put together often decides between taking on a feasible commercial project or one that loses money. It can also play a major part in deciding whether the working relationships among organizations are harmonious or dysfunctional.

Although working relationships are predominantly about people, tele-health contracts can create ambiguities in financial and service arrangements. These invariably surface later and create difficulties that can eventually play out between front-line clinical staff and patients to everyone's detriment. Misunderstanding often occurs in the courting period as contracts are agreed on. The various parties may choose to ignore these out of reticence or igno-rance, feeling they will somehow work themselves out over time. Contracts for telehealth, like all others, should never be seen as an afterthought that formalizes arrangements made earlier in the form of loose understandings and "gentlemen's agreements." These loose understandings can mask different interpretations, making tens or hundreds of thousands of dollars difference to one or other side in the contract. The contract must clearly state what is expected of whom, at what price, and how and when this will be delivered. The key to this understanding is an explicit service specification agreed on at the earliest possible stage of negotiating a contract.

SERVICE SPECIFICATIONS FOR TELEHEALTH SERVICES

No matter how small or large a telehealth project may be, a clear and detailed service specification should always be drawn up in advance of commencing the service as part of the contract. If there "is not the time to bother with this detail," repercussions usually follow, particularly if something happens to a patient. The purpose of the service specification is to define the prenuptial agreement between organizations and indicate clearly where all responsibilities lie. The precise details of any particular service specification for telehealth must depend on the exact nature of the telehealth service being provided, the health care situation in which it is to be based, and the cost of the service. Simply accepting a service specification provided by an organization as part of its original request for proposals (tendering process) is unwise. This is particularly so when developing new services to replace existing provisions using telehealth. These early service specifications are not usually robust or well enough thought through. They are rarely sufficient to use when submitting the proposal (bid), let alone to use in agreeing on a final contract.

Often when organizations put out a request proposal (tender) to deliver services, they fail to think through the fine details of how the service will be operationally delivered. With the current vogue for downsizing of management in many organizations it is not unknown to find that preliminary service specifications were drawn up by outside consultants or by people who may have since left the organization. A common reason for contracting out services to an outside organization is that they were previously badly managed within the existing organizational structure, suggesting hidden pitfalls. In practice this may also mean that there is no real in-house expertise in the organization, and the senior management team may have unrealistic expectations of what they want from their tender or request for proposals to run the service. This especially applies in telehealth, where a presentation at a conference may have caused the gleam in a senior manager's eye to build a new service. In situations like these the service specification is more than a negotiating tool. It also acts as an important communication channel.

An example of a common source of difficulty in contracting for telehealth services is the arrangement for using offices and clinics for a new service. This may seem a mundane detail in the crowded agenda of putting together complex information technology networks and clinical services, yet it is surprising how often a detail like this is forgotten. A fixation on the technological side of telehealth often means other considerations do not get the same attention to detail and can be a more expensive business to resolve than a network protocol problem. Last-minute hitches such as a leaseholder or previous provider refusing to provide vital space for the service may then surface. Problems such as needing to remove asbestos from an old building can suddenly arise when cables are installed for the network. This type of problem can be expensive to resolve in time delay and added costs, especially if the possibility has not been considered in advance and incorporated into contracting arrangements and time frames for a deadline for commencement of the service.

If the preliminary service specification provided as part of a request for proposals is poorly constructed, it should be questioned and amended in consultation with the organization putting out the contract. The process of refining a poor service specification to make it workable can be wasteful for a small telehealth service provider. It means essentially providing free consultant advice to another organization, and the small service provider has no assurance that it will eventually get the contract. If this happens, it should sound a warning bell. It means there is probably little in-house expertise in the organization putting out the contract, and the senior management team has unrealistic expectations of what they will get in the tender. Despite the monetary incentive of getting the new business it is sometimes wise to tactically withdraw from chasing a contract at an early stage. An inconsistent service specification and unrealistic budget allocation are good signs that a proposed service is undeliverable and therefore any further involvement is wasted effort.

Tables 8.9 to 8.14 cover in general terms some essential questions to consider when reviewing initial service specifications for telehealth services. These help to get an idea of the level of competency with which it has been put together. Defining each element of a service specification is important in determining the exact costs and management requirements for the service. This also determines the financial and clinical risk associated with the project. Clear costs can then be attached and a realistic bid or proposal put in for the project. An organization putting services out to tender or asking for requests for proposals gives a very clear message about its culture, competency, and credibility by how it engages in this process.

THE CONTRACT FOR TELEHEALTH SERVICES

Senior executives in telehealth organizations often view the discipline of setting down the service specification as an unnecessary complication when they are negotiating the contract. This is a common feature of health care provider organizations in general. Health care organizations often exist in a semipermanent state of crisis management and can sometimes leave comparatively junior managers to work out the exact details of a large and complex contract. This is an oversight that usually stems from a rigid distinction by the senior executive team in the organization between issues they

Table 8.9   Project Overview and General Understanding of the Market

- Does the project overview clearly summarize the service requirements and specify the parties involved, what services are being provided, and the duration of the agreement?
- Is there a clear description of the organization(s) the service is being provided for and why it is being provided? Does it detail when the service will be provided, where it will be delivered, and who will provide the premises?
- Does the specification suggest a clear understanding of the markets for telehealth, telecommunications, and clinical services, and are these realistic? Most important, does it use these to suggest revenue projections on which the eventual service will depend if it is going to survive financially?
- Are any financial data given based on real figures for providing an operational service or sales revenues? Or are they based on estimates? If they are based on estimates, is it clear how the data were derived and the confidence limits for these projections?
- What processes will the organization use to assess any bids or proposals submitted? What confidentiality agreements do they offer in the negotiating period?

consider strategic and those they consider operational. A new contract is a strategic issue for an organization. The involvement of a senior management team is usually a crucial part of the process. It is foolhardy to leave unresolved strategic considerations to be sorted out with the operational issues by a junior executive without a clear understanding of the wider implications. Organizations can suffer major financial penalties and public relations disasters through not providing the correct senior executive leadership in the contracting process.

The service specification should define the service to be provided in the final contract. This is particularly important when a telehealth service is expected to provide capitated health care services such as prison health services. The agenda driving organizations to put services such as these out to tender is saving money. If a telehealth service is to offer cost savings, it is important that the service provider defines exactly what services it is intended to pick up. Are these just routine services under expected conditions? Is there a deductible payable by the telehealth provider before access to other parts of the health care system? These considerations are vital to properly costing the service and must be done before signing a contract. When delivering health care services, the likely incidence and prevalence of disease should be factored into the projected service costs. What about meeting the costs of health care in unexpected events such as an outbreak of salmonella or a prison riot? When taking over government contracts it is important to identify areas such as this, where the preexisting service was able to tap into a wider risk pool and meet any unexpected costs. The final contract includes the fine details of finance, responsibility, and how long the service

Table 8.10   Operational Requirements for the Service

- Precisely what is the telehealth service requested and where exactly does it need to be provided? What periods of the day, week, and year is the service required for?
- Is it necessary for the service to just manage the process of remote consultation or is it to provide a clinical service? If it is to provide a clinical service, how does this fit into any wider processes of referral and care that the service may need to access?
- What are the technological components of the service, including the equipment specification? What digital data connection requirements are included in the technical specifications?
- Does the organization have a clear idea about the clinical and technical issues involved? Are they appropriate, and is there adequate expertise in house to understand these issues?
- What facilities are needed to house/deliver/manage the telehealth service being provided (e.g., clinics, office space, equipment room)? Is the organization buying the telehealth service providing some of these facilities; if so is there rent payable, and who pays for the heating, lighting, telephone, taxes, etc?
- Is the new service expected to start from one day to the next, or is there a phased introduction of the service?
- What, if any, contingency arrangements are there in case of failure of the service; who provides these and who pays? What, if any, grace period is given for backup or repair to take place in the event of a service failure?
- Which organization(s) is/are responsible for each of the components of the service that has been described? This must include whether the organization buying the telehealth service is contributing areas of the service, e.g., clinical services, LAN. If it is contributing, what are the arrangements for management of any shared facilities?
- How does the organization putting out the RFP (request for proposal) envisage that the contract will be managed? Who will monitor the contract? What are the expected standards of delivery on the contract; who will measure these and how often?
- Are there any constraints on establishing the service, e.g., referral patterns from other organizations, availability of bandwidth? If there are, how do these affect the service and payment?
- Does the telehealth service wholly manage the data networking arrangements, or does it require a shared arrangement with existing aspects of the organization's IT system?
- Is there a break clause on the contract, and what is the required period of notice?
- Who has responsibility for marketing and advertising the service?
- Who will own any intellectual property associated with the service, e.g., hardware configuration, software systems, clinical protocols?

is provided. If the service specification is well thought out and the telehealth service provider is clear about the operational service to be delivered, the final contract is usually a straightforward process.

The situation becomes more complex when a consortium arrangement provides services. Financial, operational service delivery, management, and risks for each party have to be defined. Again, it is imperative that a clear service specification, with service-level agreements among the parties in the consortium, be worked out in advance of the contract.

Table 8.11   Financial, Billing, and Contract Monitoring Considerations

* How are the telehealth services to be paid for? Is it fee-for-service, or cost and volume?
* What exactly is payable under the contract—clinical services, facilities costs, management costs?
* Are there any proposed limitations on the levels of delivering the service after which there are renegotiation clauses, e.g., upper limits/lower limits after which any of the prices paid are altered?
* How will the service be paid for—in advance or in arrears?
* How often will payments be made and in what currency (if an international service)? What, if any, arrangements are made for an inflation uplift in the price of the service each financial year?
* What are the information reporting requirements for managing and billing the service? Who will provide this information and how often?
* Are there special situations in which the service will be used, e.g., disaster management? If so, who manages these elements? Are there extra payments, or is this expected as part of the service?
* What penalties are envisaged on either side in the event of a breach of contract?
* Has the organization included a set of its audited accounts with the specification and a statement of assets?

WHAT IS NOT USUALLY INCLUDED
IN A TELEHEALTH CONTRACT

The nature of health care systems is that the interests of patients are not usually negotiated directly in the contract. Health care purchasers nominally act on the patient's behalf. A paradox of this situation is how very tangible benefits to patients are often not included in health care contracts. A great benefit of telehealth to patients is in reducing their traveling to hospitals and the need for a hospital stay. These savings in time and money to patients do not necessarily factor into the economics of telehealth contracting.

In health services development work the contract can be a creative device to use in shaping new services. The creative contracting necessary to develop telehealth provides opportunities to create benefits for patients also.

CONTRACTING FOR TELEHEALTH
AND Y2K PREPAREDNESS

Of particular concern in developing telehealth contracts for services and equipment specifications has been considerations around the problem of computers and Y2K.

The American Medical Association (AMA) ran a particularly useful series of seminars covering the issues related to Y2K and identified what it saw as

Table 8.12   Risk Management and Clinical Indemnity

- What arrangements are envisaged for backup, risk management, and disaster recovery for the service?
- Who is responsible for any clinical indemnity needed to cover the telehealth service?
- Are there set quality standards the service is expected to comply with, e.g., ISO 6000 or clinical quality standards?
- Are there clinical audit and outcomes measurement requirements, and if so who owns the data?
- Is the service year 2000 compliant, and have the necessary indemnities been covered?

the profound implications this has for health care. By extension, Y2K directly affects telehealth. The AMA has attempted to define a "Standard of Care" for dealing with the Y2K problem and for physicians and hospitals to use to ensure the safety of care to patients after the end of the year 1999.

A standard of care is an important step in trying to define the legal liability (civil and criminal) of hospitals and physicians if they fail to take adequate corrective action to protect patients. Unfortunately, it seems that a host of lawyers is preparing to bring suits against physicians and hospitals who have not been Y2K-compliant or have not ensured that they have documented due diligence in pursuing a Y2K standard of care.

Some of the areas directly specific to telehealth to consider include

- The functional integrity of personal computers and computer networks
- Biomedical devices
- Information systems
- Software applications
- Pagers used to access staff for telehealth consultations
- Remote monitoring of devices, e.g., pacemakers, infusion pumps
- HCFA and billing for services
- The integrity of digital networks used in telehealth

Table 8.13   Human Resource Considerations

- Are there any contractual requirements that staff from the preexisting service are offered employment by the telehealth service provider, e.g., European Economic Community labor laws?
- If any redundancy payments must be made to staff that the new service may be contractually obliged to inherit, who is responsible for these?
- Are there any particular requirements for staff, e.g., clinicians of a particular grade?
- Are there any pension arrangements or staff benefit requirements for the new service to take over?
- What are the training and education requirements? Who will provide these, and who will pay?
- Are equal opportunities explicitly stated in the specification?

Table 8.14   Legal Considerations

- Is it stated where the company/organization is legally registered?
- Have any laws that may govern the standards for the provision of a telehealth service, e.g., data protection, state licensure, licensing of premises been thought of and included?
- On what or whose authority in the company or organization is the request for proposals being put out?

To help protect against legal liability, telehealth providers should investigate all areas of concern. For biomedical devices everything possible to find out about the reliability of devices must be done. The onus for this should not be left to the equipment suppliers. The telehealth provider must contact all the various vendors for written assurance about Y2K reliability and document these steps. The FDA's Web site (www.FDA.gov) is a source of information. From there information can be downloaded about biomedical devices. The FDA now has a list of devices that are definitely not Y2K-compliant or reliable and is constantly updating this Web site.

Information such as this should be filed in a "Due Diligence" file. Almost all vendors now have Web sites devoted to providing information about the Y2K reliability of their products and devices. Keep revisiting these sites. Some vendors who previously certified their devices as being Y2K-compliant have subsequently altered their position. Vendors are expected to file quarterly information returns with the Securities and Exchange Commission (SEC), which now includes Y2K compliance. The SEC Web site is another information resource. Vendors should provide complete and detailed documentation to outline the steps they went through to determine that their device was Y2K-compliant. A simple assurance of Y2K compliance is not enough.

Telehealth providers must have had a Y2K strategy in place. Linked to this strategy should be detailed records of conversations, decisions, and the Y2K project plan and its implementation. Some hospitals decided that elective surgery scheduled for the first 2–3 weeks of the year 2000 either be completed earlier in 1999 or delayed until later in the year 2000 and that routine admission of patients be curtailed during the same period. This planned disruption to services will affect telehealth providers. Because of the likelihood of disruptions taking place, telehealth providers should have had contingency plans ready to put into operation on January 1, 2000. These contingency plans should have considered the people processes necessary to substitute for a breakdown in usual service provision. Planning for the problem should extend beyond the immediate considerations of the health care facility. What had to be done if power delivery systems and digital data connections fail?

9

The Business of Telehealth

Many telehealth programs seem unsure that they are in business; and if they are sure they are in business, they may be unclear about exactly what business they are in. This is a big mistake in health care systems, where health care markets are the mechanism deciding whether or not to incorporate telehealth. This reality means that, like it or not and whether they recognize it or not, all telehealth projects are ultimately in the business of telehealth if they are going to survive in the long term. Worldwide, 90% of telehealth activity currently takes place in grant-funded projects. The painful reality for the majority of telehealth projects is that they will have to consider becoming, at some stage of their lives, a commercial proposition if they are going to survive. To become a feasible proposition as a commercial provider of telehealth, existing telehealth projects and commercial start-up telehealth companies must first be clear about what part of the business of telehealth they are actually in.

For convenience and consistency we will refer to both grant-funded telehealth projects trying to become commercial ventures and start-up telehealth companies as "telehealth programs." We see each facing remarkably similar problems, except they come at them with different legacies and from different perspectives. Each is trying to find a stream or streams of revenue from telehealth activity to sustain them in the future. A grant-funded telehealth project often starts with the advantages of actually having an infrastructure in place to deliver an operational telehealth service, of having already established a name for themselves, and of having a reputation of being able to "do" telehealth. They usually start with the disadvantage of not having the lean and mean mentality a commercial stimulus brings, and this may be reflected in bloated and poorly structured processes. This does not mean that grant-funded telehealth projects are not highly efficient; they may be very effective clinically and technically, but their costs may make them commercially unsustainable.

Commercial start-up telehealth companies usually have the advantage of being clearly focused on finding a profit margin from the services they provide. They use this hunt for a profit margin to refine their product and generate revenue projections for their business plan. This helps them to start with a clean organizational slate from which to construct their business plan. Commercial start-up telehealth companies usually have the disadvantage of having little or no experience in the field unless they recruit people with existing telehealth experience onto their management team to give them this credibility.

In this chapter we look at what we call the business of telehealth and at how telehealth programs should focus on taking advantage of telehealth markets to make these large enough to sustain them. We see the development of these markets as having three major evolutionary phases. The first phase is the sale of equipment. The second is the development of a telehealth business network. The third is the sale of health care products, using the equipment and networks when the previous two are in place. To take advantage of these opportunities, telehealth companies have to be very clear about what products and services they are in the business to deliver and how they will then market and deliver these in practice.

WHAT IS THE BUSINESS OF TELEHEALTH?

In the first chapter of this book we admitted to a laissez-faire approach in how we define telehealth. We deliberately take this approach because the commercial opportunities for providing remote health care often lie between the cracks of the rigid academic style definitions used to describe terms "telemedicine" and "telehealth." With this in mind we acknowledge up front that we cannot define exactly and inclusively what is the business of telehealth. It is something dynamic and is determined by how entrepreneurial people find ways to make money from the use of information technology systems to complement or substitute for direct face-to-face contacts in the delivery of health care services. Table 9.1 shows some of the wide variety of telehealth activities a business model based on the above description has so far produced.

Table 9.1   Current Areas of Telehealth Business Activity

• Patient–practitioner consultation
• Practitioner–practitioner consultation
• Clinical investigations in health care
• Remote monitoring of patients
• Remote diagnosis in health care
• Remote treatment in health care
• The facilities management of remote health care services
• Providing information to patients
• Providing continuing education to health care practitioners
• The transfer of information throughout health care services

---

We see the business of telehealth as being defined by whatever a telehealth program can engage in profitably. Each telehealth program must therefore decide the business of telehealth in its own terms if it is going to survive. To put it bluntly, if it is going to survive, a telehealth program must have a sound business plan, an ability to implement it, and an instinct to survive.

A clear understanding of the business of telehealth therefore means looking at telehealth companies and asking them about themselves and what they are doing. A degree of introspection from telehealth programs about themselves is healthy because it helps them focus on the type of organization they are; however, some telehealth programs, especially those that have been grant-funded, seem to use a process of introspection to try to define their business. This process can pervade management meetings. The telehealth programs then become obsessive, with more time spent worrying about "who we are," "what we are," and "where we are," than on the telehealth product they are trying to market and sell. The difference between a telehealth program being an "obsessor" or a "nonobsessor" is usually dictated by whether or not it has a clear business plan to revisit and revise.

To be successful a telehealth program must have a product or products they can sell in sufficient quantities to sustain their business. The main information needed from a telehealth program to understand its business is "What is their product?" and "Can they produce and sell this at sufficient volumes to make them sustainable in the long term?" After this any "who are we," "what are we," and "where are we" considerations have relevance and context, because these can then feed into defining structures and processes within the organization, helping decide its strategic direction and business plan.

In some telehealth programs business planning seems as welcome as a bad smell at a dinner party. The business planning process is something they have tried to avoid, ignore, or neuter. Programs doing this are usually so busy doing what they want to do that they do not want to spend time looking at whether any of this activity is actually *worth* doing. Breaking into this cycle of denial can be threatening for very obvious reasons. Except for masochists, the least painful way to do this is often to focus on the product of the telehealth program. After having done this, then work backward and let the questions logically flow. Is the program profitable? What is being produced? By whom? How? This circumnavigation works because it is asking the telehealth program to look outside itself and discover what it is trying to do. The "who they are," "what they are," and "where they are" come later. Suddenly, a business plan makes sense for the first time, and the previous bad smell is recognized as a fresh rose.

We passionately believe in the need for a business plan in telehealth. This should not be a dry, irrelevant document or a chore that is performed only to please the full board or to attract outside investment. The business plan must have *passion*. The business plan describes the raison d'être for a business. Although word-processing and binding it may be a chore, the content and the process of getting agreement should have passion. What is the difference between the companies in industry that survive and those that don't with almost identical products? The answer is passion for what they are doing. Good management generates passion. Before returning to the business planning process and seeing what this passion means, what are the products of telehealth programs?

A TELEHEALTH BUSINESS'S PRODUCTS DEFINE ITS TELEHEALTH BUSINESS AREA

Many telehealth programs are clearly unsure what product it is they are trying to sell. Are they primarily in business to be an equipment vendor, a health care provider, a facilities management company for remote health care, or are they all three? Telehealth programs often represent a ragbag of competencies without defining their core business. We firmly believe the business of telehealth relates first and foremost to the delivery of care to patients, not to the technology. We always start by considering the eventual customer—the patient—when looking at a telehealth program's products. A manufacturer of specialist telehealth cameras once commented that it seemed illogical to him to take this approach: "My business is making cameras, and I will leave the care of the patients to the doctors." He was planning to expand his business into telehealth. The success of his business depended ultimately on the demand for teledermatology. He came around to the idea of the patient importance when he considered the following points:

- No matter how good he personally felt the optics of the camera were, if the dermatologist could not get the color differentiation she/he wanted to make a reliable clinical diagnosis, then it was no-sale.
- If the external illumination arrangements and camera cable made the patient uncomfortable and complaining to the practitioner at the remote end, it was also no-sale.
- The volume of teleconsultations and the likely demand in the short and medium terms for teledermatology informed him about the level of investment his company should be considering to support the new telehealth side of the business.

Whichever way we look at it the business of telehealth, it is ultimately related to the volume of telehealth transactions taking place. In any financial analysis this is where any revenue calculations have to start for a business case. In the short term a telehealth equipment supplier may sell a number of telehealth systems. The growth and expansion of the longer-term market for their equipment depends on the systems they sell being used for telehealth consultations and thereby stimulating further demand for their products. There is no greater deterrent to the sales of telehealth technology than unused equipment gathering dust in the corner of an outpatient consulting room. It is as though the equipment has a large neon sign pointing toward it, flashing the words "white elephant."

A successful teleconsultation service in any specialty depends on everybody involved in the project being figuratively in the room with the practitioner and the patient and working to make sure that the consultation is a success. Everybody in the telehealth program has a stake in having the video consultation work for the patient and the practitioner. We include a discussion of the doctor-patient relationship in this book because we feel it is important for nonpractitioners to understand the dynamics of this relationship on which the success of telehealth is so dependent. Conversely, our inclusion of this chapter about the business of telehealth is to give practitioners an understanding of the commercial support needed for a telehealth program's success. Successful telehealth programs must be able to network and for individuals within it to work as a team engaged in delivering health care services.

As I was traveling home from visiting an overseas telehealth program where the morale was low, a recent chance case comparison arose during the airplane flight that illustrates these issues. The passenger in the adjacent seat recently bought a chocolate factory, and he talked about his success in turning his company around. He had motivated the company, from production workers to night security guards, to be concerned about the taste, texture, and appearance of the chocolates. He described how as a leader he had communicated his passion to create great chocolate and overcame the apathy and cynicism. He concentrated on teamwork. Success for the company came after the whole workforce focused on the product and the customer instead of on themselves. His story contrasted with the belief in telehealth as a product to improve people's health in the academic medical center I had just visited. Here the main problem was dysfunctional relationships between different professional groups and managers. A telehealth program was being introduced into an organization at absolute loggerheads with itself. Patients were not considered at all in the cycles of repetitive arguments about turf wars and what process belonged where. The point of mentioning this anecdote is not because the message is new. Concentrating on the customer is common fare in modern management theory. The point is to illustrate the difference in the emotional climate between the health care organization and the chocolate factory—visiting an organization with a constant air of tension and hearing what cannot be done and then several hours later hearing what *can* be done. Isn't this paradoxical? Health care seems intuitively much more important than chocolate.

Let's return to the patient and what can be done. The first piece to find when dissecting the core business of a telehealth program is an understanding of how it contributes to the care of patients when a telehealth product is offered instead of conventional health care practice. If the telehealth program is a group of radiologists who are offering remote x-ray reporting facilities, their core business is a clinical service—diagnostic radiology. The contribution they make to patient care is to directly influence patient management. They must be sure they can do this at a cost and quality that is competitive. It is no good for this group of radiologists to just approach hospitals to offer their services if there are no facilities to digitally transmit x-rays for remote reporting in these hospitals. This group of radiologists must find a route to market for their product. To do so they either have to supply equipment to digitize x-rays or develop a collaborative alliance with an equipment supplier who can work with them to provide and maintain the x-ray equipment. It is of little good for the hospitals to have the x-ray equipment and the radiologists to have the expertise to read x-rays if the facility to carry the data between the two organizations is not available. This means either the hospital with the digitizing equipment must arrange this service or the group of radiologists must set up the data communication channel.

Retracing the possibilities, a group of radiologists whose prime expertise is in reporting x-rays can find they are managing a complex telehealth organization, including teleradiology equipment supply, digital service provision, and x-ray reporting, to get a route to market for their product. Some, but not all, telemedicine programs see themselves as providing the whole range of services as in the above teleradiology example. Many see that they have a "core" area of business and need to work in partnership/collaboration with other organizations to develop a secure route to market. Some telehealth programs see their role as being providers of routes to market and so work as facilities management companies to facilitate the delivery of remote health care services.

In summary, the business of telehealth is defined by the products of telehealth programs and by the network of relationships needed to produce, market, and sell these products. A telehealth program must have a business planning process and produce a business plan to detail these products and relationships in a cohesive way to generate revenue. For the business planning process to work effectively the business plan must be generated in collaboration with a range of staff from all levels of a telehealth program. This ensures that it influences the culture and behavior of the organization.

THE BUSINESS PLAN FOR A TELEHEALTH ORGANIZATION

The wide diversity of health care activity offers many fertile possibilities for developing business opportunities in telehealth. Despite this breadth of opportunity an attractive business case for a telehealth application is rarely clear-cut. Frequently, enthusiasm for the idea of using telehealth in a particular clinical setting is mistaken for having found a self-evident telehealth application. Even before making a financial analysis, the critical first step in determining whether an intended telehealth application makes good business sense is to assess whether it can successfully substitute for existing ways of delivering care. Factors to consider in making such an initial outline assessment of the business potential are included in Table 9.2.

Telehealth business opportunities are found wherever there are people willing to use this technology to generate revenue. Revenue generation from telehealth is generally accomplished in one of four main ways:

- A supplier of telehealth equipment
- A health care provider that uses telehealth to deliver services
- A facilities management service for telehealth applications
- A research and development organization for new telehealth products

The business plan links the products produced and the revenues expected from telehealth to the relationships that must be built inside and outside to manage and sustain the company. A suggested outline for a business case is included below. This outline is intended for internal purposes in the

**Table 9.2   Factors to Include in Making an Initial Assessment
of the Business Case for Telehealth**

- Is telehealth acceptable to the groups of patients and practitioners that will be expected to use it?
- Is there a natural logic to using telehealth in place of existing methods for delivering health care services?
- Will telehealth fit with the existing processes for delivering care, or can these be adapted to make it fit?
- Is the technology required adequate and sufficiently robust for the health care situation proposed for its use?
- Are there professional, legal, legislative, or regulatory constraints to using telehealth in the health care situation being targeted for its use?
- Will the introduction of telehealth fit the clinical and managerial culture in which it will be used?
- Is the area in which the telehealth application is being considered under threat and hoping to use telehealth to bolster an untenable situation?
- Is there the physical space available that will be required for operating telehealth services?
- Is there the access to capital to fund an investment in telehealth and then a clear understanding of where there is revenue potential to sustain the use of this equipment?

---

organization and to attract outside investment into the program. The outline is a template to integrate a telehealth business plan into the general business planning process. We have not included exhaustive details of the whole business planning process in this chapter. Our intention is to show how the business plan links to telehealth. Usually, someone in a telehealth organization already has experience in developing a general business plan. Before writing their own business plan we expect that a telehealth program's staff will want to consult with somebody having this expertise and look through the many books available on writing business plans. We are not going to suggest any particular books. This is a matter of personal preference best determined by browsing in a bookshop or visiting an on-line book vendor.

A BUSINESS PLAN FOR A
TELEHEALTH SERVICE PROVIDER

1. An Outline of the Telehealth Company
    - A summary of the company in terms of length of time in existence and whether a limited company
      - What is the annual revenue of the company?
      - How many employees are there in the company?
      - How widely nationally and internationally does/will it sell its products?

- Major affiliations of the company with hospitals, other health care organizations, telecommunications companies, etc., necessary for it to deliver its services
- Names and titles of shareholders and directors of the company, with a short history of when, why, and how it was founded
- An outline of the executive team and the structure of the company with an organizational chart

2. The Business of the Telehealth Company
   - What are the principal products that the company produces—goods or services—and what if anything makes the products of the company unique?
   - An outline of the principal customers, or projected customers for the telehealth products the company produces:
     - Why are they or why will they be customers?
     - What is it about the company's products or business relationships that attracts or will attract these customers?
   - What are the annual sales or annual projected sales of the company's products, e.g., the number of teledermatology, teleradiology transactions per year?
     - What is the income expected for each product?
   - Are the products solely provided by the telehealth company or are goods and services from other sources, e.g., telcos, packaged into the products?
   - Are the sales of the telehealth company's products dependent on particular factors such as subsidies, grants, or the existence of structural features of health care such as purchasing and providing of health care in the United Kingdom and HMOs in the United States?
   - Are the products of the company dependent on particular staff or relationships, e.g., is the teledermatology based on the reputation of a particular individual and his/her unique characteristics?
   - Are the sales of the company's products dependent on a short-term shortage in the market, e.g., will building a new local hospital obviate the need for remote health and affect the company's market?

3. Arrangements for the Production of the Company's Products
   - How and where are the products of the company produced or provided in the case of services?
   - The process for the strategic management of operational services and the flexibility of the telehealth company to increase or decrease the amount of its production
   - What are the changes to the cost profiles of the products from these changes?

- How is the production process managed, e.g., what is the process for booking and arranging telehealth transactions? Are there wide fluctuations for telehealth transactions from week to week or month to month?
- Is there a waiting list for the products or surplus capacity, e.g., are there usually empty teleconsultation appointments or do patients have to book in advance and wait?
- Who provides the clinical services? Physicians? Nurses? Who else? Who employs these practitioners and what are the contractual relationships for their employment?
- Who provides the technical and support services such as network manager, secretarial, etc.? What are the contractual arrangements for their employment?
- What are the costs per telehealth transaction broken down into the direct costs of the care aspect of the service and the overhead costs?
- Are there any bonus or incentive schemes? Are staff members of professional organizations and trade unions?
- What are the trends in recruitment and pay settlements that may affect the telehealth company and its ability to provide services?

4. Quality Measures for Telehealth Products and Clinical Research and Development
   - Clinical audit of telehealth services. What is the size of program? Frequency of program audit and the percentage of the services that are subject to audit? The size of budget for this program? The number of services not meeting quality standards annually?
   - Clinical outcome measurements
   - Clinical research and development programs

5. Clinical Risk Management, Claims Management, and Clinical Indemnity
   - A description of the clinical risk management program for telehealth. The size of the program? The annual budget? The percentage of the services covered? The audit program's relationship with other health care organizations?
   - What number of adverse incidents occur per year and in what areas of the telehealth's provision of care? What is the comparison with past years and how does it benchmark with other telehealth companies?
   - Is the telehealth company liable for clinical negligence? If so, how is clinical negligence cover provided? What is the annual premium for clinical negligence cover? What are the deductibles and ceilings applicable to any clinical negligence indemnity?
   - What is the number, if any, of clinical negligence claims per year? The number of current claims for clinical negligence? The anticipated size

of any financial settlements for clinical negligence? The financial call on the company, if any for clinical negligence?

- What is the process for managing clinical complaints?
- What are the procedures for clinical claims?
- Are there any clinical claims outstanding against the organization?

6. Sales and Marketing of Telehealth Products
   - How are the telehealth products marketed and sold? What are advertising costs, conferences display costs, journal article costs? Where are the products of the company marketed, and why are these areas targeted?
   - The sales and marketing force—people employed?
   - Marketing and sales of telehealth products through the Internet as a sales and marketing medium?
   - Annual budget for sales and marketing?
   - What is the size of the telehealth market for the company?
   - What is the sales potential for the company? What is realistic? What is achievable?
   - How are customer preferences and satisfaction measured?

7. Competition in the Telehealth Market an Future Market Trends
   - Who are the company's major competitors?
   - What are the prices of the company in comparison to its competitors for the range of products provided?
   - What are the relative market placings and why?
   - What are probable future trends in products, and how will these affect the position of the company vis-à-vis the competition?
   - What are the strengths, weaknesses, opportunities, and threats to the telehealth company in the short/medium/long-term future?
   - What share of the telehealth market does the company receive compared to its competition?
   - How may the activity of government, including governments in other countries, affect the telehealth market?
   - Have the telehealth products of the company been reviewed in journals? If so, does evidence exist for the effectiveness of the products?

8. Management of the Telehealth Company
   - What is the organizational structure of the company?
   - Does the telehealth company rely on in-house management expertise, or does it contract out as required?
   - What are the salaries of the board of directors and senior management, and are the remuneration packages decided?
   - How is the board chosen and what are the various board committees?
   - Who is the company secretary?

9. Financial Position of the Company and Financial Management
   - Arrangements for independent audit?
   - Arrangements for internal audit?
   - Arrangements for company ledger?
   - Arrangements for standing financial instructions?
   - Short-term financial plan?
   - Long-term financial plan?
   - Arrangements for financial reporting?

10. Company's Equity Capitalization and Debt
    - Type of company: PLC, limited company, corporation?
    - Major shareholders?
    - Capital assets?
    - Capitalization and where this is held?
    - Creditors?

11. Research and Development
    - Annual spending on R&D?
    - Arrangements for R&D strategy and new product development?
    - Future predictions for the effects of evidence-based practice on telehealth?
    - Future predictions for the impact of new technology on telehealth provision?
    - Future funding plan for R&D?

10

The Management of Telehealth Programs

As physicians who have moved from directly providing care into the very different cultures of management and policy development in health care services, we see the way telehealth is evolving as a melting pot in which many of the current challenges for health care organizations are being played out. Maybe this convergence and mix of culture, management, and policy issues attracted us to work in telehealth development in the first place. The future of telehealth seems no more uncertain to us than any other sector of health care in these turbulent times. Telemedicine gurus have different opinions about what will be the single most critical factor in determining telehealth's success. Some telehealth experts suggest it will be the cost of the technology; others say it will be the cost and availability of bandwidth, and still others think it will be the acceptance of telehealth by clinicians. We believe, above all else, that the quality of management in telehealth programs will be a decisive factor in determining the future success and survival of telehealth programs.

In stressing how important we feel the management of telehealth programs will be, we are stating what is obvious. We do not see any one overriding factor holding the key to the future of telehealth. Its future depends on how an array of problems are managed in a structured and ordered way over time. Because the health care environment is so changeable, this management process must be flexible to accommodate altered circumstances and to deliver set objectives on time. Setting these deliverables means projects must be based on a strategic plan. In turn, making this strategic plan happen

216

requires structures and processes to be put in place within a culture that applies them coherently. To some people what we have written is blindingly obvious. To others it is fuzzy talk from the distrustful breed called managers. The truth lies in what delivers, not in words.

In this chapter we look at how the culture of a telehealth program and the subsequent management (or nonmanagement) of structure and process may affect the eventual outcome of projects. In the end the success of an organization is judged on what it is able to deliver, not on the good intentions with which it started out. Look at how the general industrial and commercial sectors in the United Kingdom and the United States have adapted and moved on from dysfunctional times in the 1970s and 1980s. Their problems were similar in nature to many that currently beset health care. Industry and commerce succeeded through adopting management principles that health care organizations still seem to have problems understanding and applying.

HOW CULTURE DETERMINES STRATEGIC THINKING AND THE DIRECTION OF A TELEHEALTH PROGRAM

Whether a telehealth program is a separate organization or a part of a larger and more complex health care organization, its culture usually differs from the general culture of most health care organizations. The nature of telehealth is about networks, networks of people and information technology networks. Organizations based on the principle of networking do not work well in central "command and control" modes of management. Command-and-control structures are often wasteful and inefficient of time and resources. Networking organizations work well with delegated authority and devolved power structures, where people have clear roles and responsibilities and work according to agreed-on policies and procedures to define areas in which they have agreed autonomy.

In contrast to the devolved organization a typical health care organization such as a hospital has a hierarchical structure. Hospitals are usually managed in a central command-and-control mode, where operational decision-making responsibility is retained at a high level in the organization. If a networking organization works closely with a command-and-control organization and each fails to make the adjustments for the cultural differences, then the results are like the proverbial chalk and cheese or oil and water. They just do not mix well. It is not a good solution for a telehealth organization to try to adopt a command-and-control structure. Although it may help in the working relationship with the health care organization, it hinders other important relationships. There are three possible "cultural mixes" when a command-and-control organization (e.g., a hospital) and a networking organization (e.g., a telehealth program) try to work together. These cultural mixes are shown diagrammatically in Figure 10.1.

Many effective managers in devolved organizations that network successfully would agree that a quick way to read the "cultural temperature" of an organization they visit (e.g., a telehealth program) is to ask at different levels of that organization, "Does the organization have a mission statement?" Then a supplementary "Do they know what the values of the organization are?" In some health care organizations a typical response within the organization to this question is the cynical reply "Any organization with time for mission statements when there are things to get on with has problems." We read the reaction of "no mission statement" or "mission statement and values not known in the organization" as indicating that the organization is either in command-and-control mode or aimless.

We use the presence of the mission statement as an initial indication of whether the organization has a clear purpose people believe in and of a set of values to bind the organization together. Lack of a mission and values suggests that the organization is probably dysfunctional in today's rapidly changing world. It is dysfunctional because the organization probably has no agreed-to purpose and no coherence of effort. On further acquaintance it may become clear that the organization is incapable of defining a strategy or implementing operational policies. The management of a telehealth organization has to start with the culture, mission, and purpose of the telehealth organization. The permutations and combinations of telehealth organization are too many to give any one prescription for how the organization should be structured. We will cover only the broad process issues that apply.

If the telehealth program is a separate and autonomous organization, then its own board should agree on the mission and values of the organization in collaboration and consultation with the staff. If the telehealth organization is part of a larger health care organization, it should agree on its own mission and values that must be compatible with the wider organization in which it operates. The function of the senior-level tier of management in the organization is to define the strategic direction of the organization in conjunction with its staff. Although a telehealth program may have only a few staff and managers, small numbers of people do not prevent this process from happening.

The senior management tier is responsible for defining operational policies and setting objectives to deliver the strategic aims of the organization. People in health care often forget the important process of clearly defining roles and responsibilities for everybody in the organization and developing clear policies and procedures for communication. These processes may seem

1. Cultural mix of telehealth organization with *no* devolved management structure for networking working with a central command-and-control health care organization

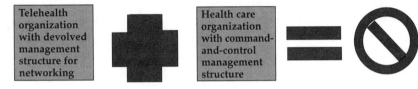

2. Cultural mix of telehealth organization with devolved management structure for networking working with central command-and-control health care organization where each is not aware of nor sensitive to the management culture of the other

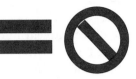

3. Cultural mix of telehealth organization with devolved management structure for networking working with central command-and-control health care organization where each is not aware of nor sensitive to the management culture of the other

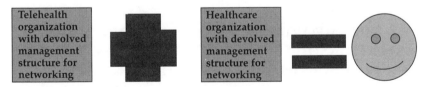

Figure 10.1   Cultural mix of telehealth and health care organization.

laborious, but they are important to establish if the organization is going to perform in a coordinated manner. The derivation of the concept strategy is from an ancient Greek sea victory over the Persians. Although the Persian fleet was stronger, with much larger and more powerful ships, the Greeks lured them into a cove. In the cove the smaller Greek ships acted in consort and outmaneuvered the Persian fleet and so defeated them. The advantage for a telehealth organization of being small and maneuverable is the ability to adapt rapidly and deal with change.

Another important aspect of managing a networking organization such as a telehealth program with a devolved management structure is staff recruitment. Clear job descriptions and personnel specifications must be prepared in advance. These make explicit the roles and responsibilities of any new people recruited into the organization. It used to be a guiding principle of recruitment into health care to check to see if potential hires had followed a linear trajectory as their careers progressed. Now this style of recruitment is often a mistake. People who have had linear career paths are often rigid and inflexible in their approach to problem solving. It is essential when undertaking development work in a rapidly changing environment such as telehealth to have people working on the program who are adaptable, innovative, and proactive.

The picture we are beginning to paint as a model for a telehealth organization is in many ways the antithesis of a traditional health care organization. These traditional health care organizations used to be ideal for professionals to work in for the very reason that they changed only slowly and even then after great deliberation. The medical director is a vital figure in the changing health care environment. The medical director in a telehealth organization can be clinical and nonclinical (managerial). The management role involves responsibilities such as those shown in Table 10.1.

The different culture can make it easier if a telehealth program does not directly employ physicians itself. Physician employment can remain with the collaborating health care organizations (e.g., hospitals), and their clinical relationship with the telehealth organization can then be defined by a service-level agreement.

THE IMPORTANCE OF ESTABLISHING GOOD RELATIONSHIPS WITH DOCTORS TO DEVELOPING SUCCESSFUL TELEHEALTH PROGRAMS

Whether a telehealth program employs its own doctors or works closely with doctors in other health care organizations, good relationships with its doctors are vital. The external criteria of success for a telehealth program are often judged in terms of the number of patient referrals they attract.[185] Typically, patient data collected by telehealth programs includes the numbers of

+ Consultations undertaken
+ Radiographs read
+ Pathology slides reported
+ Diagnoses made

**Table 10.1   The Nonclinical Responsibilities of a
Medical Director in a Telehealth Program**

- Clinical audit and clinical outcomes measurement
- Clinical protocol development
- Clinical contracting
- Clinical risk management
- Claims management
- Managing research and development
- Professional development

These data are used as performance measures to assess the progress of a telehealth program and form the basis for gauging the revenue stream in fee-for-service contracts. Patient referrals to telehealth programs are usually through direct referral from doctor to doctor[111] or nurse practitioner to doctor.[93] How well a telehealth program performs is therefore directly related to the clinical practice of physicians who refer patients to it. Productive and functional collaborations with the clinicians referring patients are therefore crucial elements to achieving success for any telehealth project/program.[186]

One of the roles for physicians in health care settings is to act as gatekeepers who decide the onward care and referral pathways for patients. Physicians have the technical knowledge and the professional power to attract or block patient referrals into telehealth projects. Presence or absence of their support is therefore a critical success factor for any telehealth program. Support for a telehealth program from physicians may be needed at all levels of a health care organization, including the board, senior executive team, directorate managers, clinical and scientific advisors, and front-line clinicians. However, the seniority of the clinician in the health care hierarchy is no gauge of his/her relative importance to a project's success. Full support from an organization's medical director may not compensate for lack of support from front-line clinical staff if it is they who are required to make the day-to-day patient referrals on which the program's survival depends.

Professional Hierarchies and the
Development of Telehealth Programs

Health care systems are typical hierarchies, and this makes introducing new technology such as telehealth difficult to manage. A wide range of practitioners within health care organizations can raise professional barriers and block the progress of a telehealth project. Ways of working with physicians and other health care professionals to successfully "change manage" the introduction of new projects such as telehealth are poorly researched. We have therefore had to look at the experience of organizations in industries outside health care with similar professional hierarchies to develop strategies for working with physicians to manage change.

A tried and tested strategy from industry to use in changing the work practice of professionals involves building three groups of organizational bridges to support taking a new development forward.[187] These three bridges can be broadly classified into three types: procedural, human, and organizational; they are outlined in Table 10.2.

Managing Relationships with Doctors in Telehealth Programs

A telehealth program or project may be clinically relevant, fully funded, technically perfect, and project-planned down to the last iota of detail. Nevertheless, it can fail without buy-in of key participants. Among the usual cast list of players, the most problematical group to sell a project to is often the physicians. Objections raised by physicians to a project vary from the theoretical and ethical to the practical and technical. Sometimes these objections may even seem petty given the professional status that doctors enjoy. Opposition from one or more of the medical staff can surface unexpectedly and at any stage, from the initial planning phase to that of the fully operational service.

Fear of change is a common reason for this reaction from physicians. Another is the cultural shock for physicians of working with an organization where there are networks rather than hierarchies and relationships are predominantly contractual rather than professional. Physicians are used to working autonomously with patients rather than contractually, of having their working relationships defined by tradition and by their professional bodies. For these reasons alone it is quite understandable that physicians find telehealth projects threatening, and this can cause them to be obstructive mainly from fear of the unknown.

Although possible, it is now much less likely that a physician will object openly and vehemently in the manner of Sir Lancelot Sprat (an archetypal surgeon in a famous series of British books by Richard Gordon, made into movies). It is much more likely that a physician's objection to a project will be for a clinical or technical reason associated with the delivery of care. What clues can help to show whether the concern a physician voices about a particular aspect of a telehealth project is prompted by giving vital technical knowledge to forward the work of the team or because she/he is undermining the project?

Table 10.2   The Three Bridges to Support Professionals in Development Projects

Procedural bridges
  • Establish joint planning groups
  • Joint staffing of projects
  • Joint evaluation/appraisal

Human bridges
  • Focus on relationships that convey information between people
  • Focus on relationships that shift responsibility from one person to another
  • Focus on interpersonal alliances and informal contacts

Organizational bridges
  • Develop project task forces
  • The use of facilitators

A popular myth is that doctors over 50 years of age are the ones most resistant to change and the most likely to reject new ideas. This myth implies that it is the clinicians who are most likely to make life difficult for new health care developments such as telehealth. This is not a consistent enough pattern to be useful in deciding who are and who are not allies. Both younger and older clinicians are capable of being obstructive as well as supportive if the situation is threatening. Older clinicians who are near retirement often feel they need not worry about "protecting territory," whereas younger clinicians feel they have a lot to lose with their working life ahead of them. Data from studies of managing professional groups in industry suggest that it is only when professionals of any age feel secure about themselves that they can face new challenges and achieve results.[188] We avoid all preconceptions about physicians, as with others related to discriminators of age, sex, ethnicity, religion, and social class. We also add another preconception to avoid—the specialty of the physician. Physicians do not necessarily follow the traditional stereotypes, particularly when they move out of role into a new project area such as telehealth.

Our preference when working with physicians or any other group (including managers) is to remain neutral and assess each person by his/her contribution to the team. This is achieved by watching how they support or hinder what the whole group is trying to achieve. We reserve judgment and work with people as they are, not how we would ideally like them to be. This is for pragmatic reasons associated with the project as well as personal concern for the individual. However people are behaving, whether they are infuriating or otherwise, it is important not to isolate them. Wherever possible these situations must be reversed. This often can be done by involving them in decision-making processes. Research shows that projects will succeed more often when there is a widespread participation in decision-making processes and when a wider group[189,190] makes final decisions. Autocratic decision-making processes may be attractive as a gut response to the challenge of getting a new program off the ground, but ultimately, we often find that the costs to the program in terms of alienating and demotivating people make any gains from this tactic illusory. A hallmark of networking organizations with devolved management structures is decision making by consensus, not at the behest of an autocratic voice of command and control.

The training of physicians is traditionally through command and control. It takes patience to work with such physicians and teach them the new skills of consensus decision making. This effort is usually very rewarding. Working in hospitals was stressful long before the added angst of the current organizational changes in health care. The stresses result from dealing with sick and dying people in need of help. When coming from the calmer world outside into stressful health care situations it is easy to make snap judgments about people, particularly doctors. Doctors currently face criticism from many sides, but any criticism often changes when a close member of the person's family needs medical help. We then appreciate that doctors often have a 24-hour-a-day, 365-day-a-year commitment, a commitment few other professionals or workers maintain. Judgments made in haste about doctors often turn out to be premature and wrong conclusions in a later analysis. For example, what may seem to be an intolerant, unappreciative, or negative comment heard in the pressure to roll out a program may nonetheless be a voice of reason. It may be the only warning that a telehealth program's strategy is unclear, incorrect, insensitive, or poorly marketed. In this situation the price of pride, oversensitivity, and a snap judgment against a critical voice can be the loss of an important collaborator at best and at worst can mean harm to patients and the failure of the program.

How to Work Effectively with Doctors on Project Management/Steering Groups

By their very nature project groups can become unfocused, particularly if they have no clear strategy. If the lack of focus continues, members of the group sense that the value of the group is becoming marginal and irrelevant. When this happens, they will often drift away. When people are disengaging from a project group for this reason, they rarely admit directly to a problem. Instead they usually make excuses and then miss future meetings. Although interest in a steering group may be all-consuming for a project/program leader, the project may amount to only a small fraction of the workload of a busy doctor or senior manager who attends the group. Once these people feel a meeting is unproductive and tedious, they will usually drift away and use their time more profitably elsewhere. It is for the project leader to capture the enthusiasm of people and keep them motivated. In new projects/programs, once people have gone it is difficult to get them back and reengaged.

Physicians can find group decision making by consensus foggy and unfocused. They are often familiar with more didactic and gladiatorial processes for reaching decisions, where the loudest and most forceful usually wins. Table 10.3 gives some simple rules to help make sure steering groups containing physicians work effectively.

Finding the right balance between sensitivity and oversensitivity when working with groups is vital. Remember, all behaviors do not have to relate to the project in hand. A brusque entrance and a dissatisfied look from a physician may be a sign of a clinical or interpersonal problem facing the person elsewhere. When a steering group is in the early stages of its life, it is easy to be overly sensitive to what happens because of anxiety about the outcome of the project. If this is allowed to happen, then all sorts of outside emotional and operational baggage, often totally unrelated to the business of the group, can creep into meetings by mistake. The ability to pick up on these subtle nuances makes a skillful chairperson a windfall in the initial stages of developing a steering group for a project/program. Good chairing skills are about much more than just driving a particular business agenda forward.

A good chairperson understands the political dynamics and then works productively with these and any emotional undercurrents. It is not necessarily a cause for concern if such undercurrents exist. Complex dynamics usually go with the territory of having any group destined to achieve real results. It is far better to have a lively group driving an agenda forward than to have a group reminiscent of the undead in a horror movie. The emotional tone and the tempo of the group often need setting by the manager with the prime responsibility for taking the telehealth project forward. It is easy to fall into negativism in health care environments. A "can do" mentality must be matched by getting things done. Telehealth projects have this capacity to excite because they have in tangible results, including the sudden appearance of shiny new hardware and software linking the project to the world outside.

Managing the Impact of Telehealth on Medical Practice

Under most circumstances it is a given that telehealth projects must attract patient referrals for survival; therefore, successful and sustainable telehealth programs must de facto change existing clinical practice in a health care

Table 10.3   Suggestions for Making Steering Groups Work

- Make sure that the group is relevant. If it is not, disband and reconfigure.
- Make sure that it can make real decisions (can allocate resources).
- Set a clear agenda.
- Make sure clear notes are taken.
- Run meetings strictly to time.
- Set clear action points.
- Action individuals to do work.
- Set clear and realistic time scales for actions.
- Include in the minutes action points, person actioned, and time scale.
- Don't allow any bullying and intimidation to make decisions.

organization. Given its fundamental requirement for clinical change, how can it be a surprise that doctors, as a group, find telehealth difficult and threatening? Sudden change contradicts the comfortable professional ethos on which medicine is historically based. This ethos is invested with several thousand years of effort from its predecessors and usually somewhere between 6 and 20 years of individual professional training to instill, distill, and mature. This makes working with doctors to change clinical practice a real challenge. This challenge is often greatest of all at the beginning, when it is necessary to successfully sell a project to a group of physicians. They are usually the group with the most power to bring about the project's failure and sometimes the most to lose in terms of disruption to the traditional power structure if it succeeds.

In selling telehealth projects to physicians it may or may not help to have a project leader with a medical background. This can turn out to be either an advantage or a liability to the project, depending on individual circumstances, which depend as much on personality as on the professional and technical skill sets of the particular individuals. It is best to have a project leader who can be a chameleon and change his/her approach depending on the situation encountered. We have mentioned how management cultures differ and the need to build organizational bridges. Sometimes the best bridge is a person who is able to cross between the two cultures, communicate between them, and reassure both sides. So if they are likely to be tricky, how are relationships with doctors managed most effectively in telehealth projects when the issues at stake are effectively managing clinical change?

We believe it is always better to be proactive and anticipate situations, rather than avoid them through ignorance or choice and then face having to recapture lost ground. For example, telehealth projects should avoid at all costs starting dysfunctional relationships with physicians or physician groups. Either side can initiate the dysfunction, and a good way for a project to start this off is by "doctor bashing." Doctor bashing is currently a popular pastime. Although this is a route to vent frustrations, it is both unproductive and futile. It usually arises when two command-and-control cultures meet. The time put into developing a mission statement and values to foster a different culture may seem wasted at times but so often pays off in the long term. Groups of people who understand each other can usually work together. Groups who don't understand each other can interminably rerun old battles.

The consensus approach of the devolved networking organization can be inappropriate, especially if it results in ritually adopting a condescending maxim such as "Let's make sure we have the docs on board." In devising a strategy for a telehealth project the prime goal should be making it successful. A successful strategy takes into consideration the relative roles of all the key players and how they fit into the bigger picture of what all are trying to achieve. If it is not relevant or productive to include doctors, then there is no need to do so. If the project does not require medical involvement, it may antagonize other health care professionals to gratuitously include doctors when they are not needed.

When they are among the key players, the buy-in of medical staff to any project that involves them is vital. Often this can't be achieved straightaway. Success in the world of health services development is often relative. At times an enormous triumph may just be not facing open hostility and opposition. Buy-in is not a passive process, like waiting for ice to freeze. The words imply action—if the buy-in of a person is vital, then the project must be sold actively and persuasively. If a particular doctor or nurse is needed by a telehealth program to help it succeed, it is usually best to approach her/him honestly and then sell the program with conviction. The motivation of people in health care is usually more complex than money. Concerns about patients, status, and tradition may all play a part, so conviction must address these various driving forces. Although they are sometimes criticized, health care professionals are generally highly motivated, and they usually respond well to people with similar energy and motivation.

Success in Marketing a Telehealth Program to Doctors

To market a telehealth program to a group of physicians it is often best to start with the patient. Physicians need to know up front whether any proposed changes to practice will benefit patients and that no anticipated adverse medicolegal consequences exist. Aside from these concerns, they, like most of us, want to know if they will suffer financially or lose personal prestige.

By their nature many health service development projects involve breaking with tradition. The sense of quasi-rebellion this creates can give a new program a license to have fun. This license can then work to unlock the creativity in the most surprising people. Creative energy in health care organizations often lies dormant, sapped by hierarchical walls and stifling traditions over time. A new telehealth project/program should actively seek these untapped and often unrecognized resources and set them to work. Frequently, the physician who is most passionate in his/her initial objection to a program/project is later won around and eventually becomes its most fervent supporter. Passion swings easily. Quiet and stubborn opposition is much more heavily entrenched and is usually difficult to detect. Clinician and manager alike, there are those who can subtly block progress by being faint of heart and chronically failing to deliver on their agreed commitments. Those are the ones to watch out for.

MOTIVATING HEALTH CARE PROFESSIONALS TO WORK WITH TELEHEALTH PROGRAMS

Until very recently the idea that work could be fun in health care organizations was a heresy. That humor and health care are connected may seem anathematous (the legacy of a work ethic more concerned with dogma than deliverables?). It is the very serious and stressful side of health care that makes humor a safety valve that often needs releasing to diffuse tense situations. When the going gets tough, as it does in all projects, the value of humor is often forgotten. Part of what keeps people involved in groups, meetings, and projects is being involved with a group of people who are creative, productive, and amusing. Sensitivity is needed to match any emotion introduced to the mood prevailing in the group and whatever the current set of circumstances are. Creative solutions should accept current circumstances, and if they introduce optimism combined with fun and humor, it can motivate far more than repeated predictions of doom and gloom. Most demotivating of all is denial and to keep blindly ignoring what is obvious.

These thoughts are intuitive for most of us, and they have been shown to work. The best ways to motivate professionals and initiate creativity[191] are shown in Table 10.4. These values are very different from those usually found in most health care organizations, where management is by command and control. Although it is important for a telehealth program to be optimistic and have a can-do mentality, it is also important to be realistic. The chances of success of radically changing a health care organization by introducing a telehealth program are slim but not impossible. Part of any telehealth program's strategy must be to decide whether it is better to make the choice of a creative environment where health care professionals are

Table 10.4   Ways to Motivate Professionals

- Reward risk taking.
- Support and encourage new ideas.
- Support and encourage attempts at new methods of working.
- Avoid a pattern of communication that follows organizational lines and promotes a culture where people feel the need to cover themselves.
- Encourage reading and communications with people outside the immediate organization.
- Encourage and support nonconformity.
- Encourage joke telling and humor.
- Reward and recognize people for achievement rather than punishing failure.

enthusiastic and responsive a priority. This often means choosing an organization with a forward-thinking and enlightened managerial approach. In the current climate this environment is often found in primary care–focused organizations, those with similar devolved management structures who depend on developing networks to succeed.

USING REWARDS AND SANCTIONS IN DEVELOPING TELEHEALTH PROJECTS

In spite of a project's or program's best attempts at working openly and collaboratively, things sometimes just don't work. When these situations occur and the solution is not straightforward, it may require the artful use of either a carrot or a stick to move things forward. In health care it is often difficult to decide when and which of these modalities to use. Who is the most appropriate person to deploy them if they are needed? These judgments require people management and project management skills to make distinctions between the underlying political agendas and the serious concerns about clinical safety. These kinds of issues show what is often at stake in taking a telehealth program forward. People management skills are often not enough to manage these dilemmas in health care; another set of skills is needed. These skills help distinguish when a turn of events is passing from the realm of the technical and productive to the political and maybe even getting to the seriously dysfunctional. Recognizing these changes is often difficult when working with professional groups.

Professionals often invoke defensive positions and suggest that any proposed change will harm patients. This tactic has the effect of instantly polarizing an issue. The polarization occurs because a cardinal rule in health care is at risk of being broken. This rule states: "You must not harm patients." In effect by suggesting harm to patients a practitioner is laying a trump card onto the table. The stake is being raised (as in a big card game). Is this a bluff? Correctly reading this strategy is often crucial in the acceptance of a telehealth program, particularly if it takes place in an open meeting with other health care professionals or patients. Is the project/program being finessed so that the "Old World" prevails and an unwelcome change blocked? Or is this a genuine concern about patient welfare? Is the concern important enough to take precedence over the intended direction of the project/program? Situations like these are no longer as frustrating or as impossible to resolve as they were in the past. New management initiatives and clinical tools are now available in health care to help. Examples of these are shown in Table 10.5.

These management tools bring an element of objectivity into what were previously untenable, no-win situations. There are powerful new ways of looking at the clinical effects of changes in practice, and these management tools are now being applied in health care. If telehealth is considered potentially harmful to patients, it is now legitimate, and expected, to ask "What is the evidence for this assertion?" Is this objection raised about the project scientifically valid or is it just anecdote? These decisions-making tools allow information about outcomes of patient treatment, care delivery, and cost to be factored against any clinical objection. It is now common to evaluate new health care developments to objectively assess what their effects will be. Telehealth should be no different. Evaluations do not necessarily cost large sums of money. Powerful assessments can be done from routine data sets if they are systematically collected.

If a situation arises where judgments need to be made about any potential risks or adverse effects associated with a telehealth program, then the program must interface with clinical and general management systems in the wider health care organization in which it is operating. Concerns about clinical risk, litigation, and human resource implications may have to be aired. This organizational interface should be agreed on in the contractual relationships between a telehealth program and a health care provider through the service-level agreement. This must specify who will lead on any review and who owns any resulting data. Any rewards and sanctions will then fit into the wider management and health care delivery context in which the telehealth project is operating.

MANAGING PATIENT REPRESENTATION IN TELEHEALTH PROJECTS

Success is an elusive animal in health care development projects, and finding it usually requires a flexible approach. It means keeping in mind that

Table 10.5   Assessing the Effects of New Developments of Patient Care

- Evidence-based medicine
- Clinical audit
- Outcomes research
- Protocol-based care
- On-line data searches
- Patient focus groups

compromises can often provide something for everybody. Compromise solutions in health care must always include the patients who can be easily forgotten when issues of power, prestige, and money are at stake. Although concern for patients is often mentioned in health care meetings, the actual patients are rarely represented, much less present in person. Increasingly, patients are being asked to represent their own interests. It is both good karma and good management practice to include patients whenever their interests need discussing in telehealth development steering groups.

TELEHEALTH AND MANAGING PRACTITIONER–PATIENT RELATIONSHIPS IN THE FUTURE

We believe the future for telehealth is about developing new relationships between health care practitioners and patients. It is impossible to decide how these relationships should be developed and nurtured without an understanding of the current doctor-patient relationship. Telehealth programs must work collaboratively with doctors to develop new ways of delivering health care that overcome the deficiencies that have beset the traditional doctor-patient relationship. We currently know very little about the practitioner-patient relationship in telehealth. The absence of this explicit knowledge is not a bar to the rapid development of telehealth, and with it comes the possibility of an exploration of new practitioner-patient relationships, which should be a learning process. The interface among technology, information resources, and human interaction can then be critically evaluated.

It took 2,000 years to critically examine the traditional doctor-patient relationship. The lesson from this is not to cling to traditional models of practitioner-patient interaction because they are self-evident. Telehealth programs should look instead at developing the future relationships between clinicians and patients. The relationships and levels of understanding between doctor and patient are personal and confidential. Telehealth programs can assess the adequacy, accuracy, and humanity of practitioner-

**Table 10.6   Important Factors in Assessing the
Practitioner–Patient Relationship in Telehealth**

- Medicolegal issues and indemnity
- Clinical and managerial responsibility
- Ethical committee approval
- Informed consent of patients
- Regular project review

patient relationships in videoconsultation as part of managing the quality of their services. These assessments should be aimed at providing clear evidence of the effectiveness of teleconsultation and feedback mechanisms to improve the quality of teleconsultations. To incorporate these processes into telehealth programs, areas such as those listed in Table 10.6 should be managed by the telehealth program.

CONCLUDING THOUGHTS ON THE MANAGEMENT OF TELEHEALTH PROGRAMS

In this chapter we have looked at some of the important issues in managing telehealth programs. We have not dwelt on the management of other important technical and clinical areas that need to be managed operationally in telehealth programs. Many of these aspects are covered in other chapters of the book. The technical and clinical details of telehealth are changing and will continue to change. Many technical aspects of managing data networks and equipment will be redundant by the time this book is published. We are fascinated at the way in which the technology of telehealth is rapidly evolving. However, it is our firm belief that limitations to the expansion of telehealth are not technical nor do they have to do with the cost of equipment, although these are important issues. The major limitation to the growth of telehealth is the people issues. Telehealth is changing the ways physicians and other practitioners have traditionally delivered care and related to their patients. The success of telehealth depends on managing people as well as machines. Machines are the easy part to manage in the symbiosis between person and technology that is telehealth.

11

Choosing the Right Technology for Telehealth

The cost of buying and leasing the hardware needed to make telehealth transactions is falling dramatically, and at the same time the processing power of the equipment continues to rise. Digital data networks to connect the hardware elements needed for telehealth are rapidly expanding, and data compression algorithms further increase their capacity to transmit data. Ever-burgeoning information technology improvement makes it difficult to decide which technology best supports a telehealth program and when is the best time to invest in equipment. This race for technical innovation sometimes leads people to base judgments about the relative success of telehealth programs as much on the state of their equipment as on the quality of the operational health care services they deliver.

The choice of technology for a telehealth program and when to buy it must be based on how appropriately the equipment supports the underlying business of delivering clinical services. It can be far healthier for a telehealth program to stay with low equipment overhead costs if these make it competitive and self-sustaining, rather than blindly invest for the sake of following a fashion for new technology. If telehealth programs are seduced into taking the latter route, they can incur high overhead costs, which then have to be passed on to their consumers. Rising costs trigger a spiral in which telehealth transaction costs progressively rise. Consultation costs can then reach levels as high as $4,000–$5,000 per consultation (although these may never pass on as actual costs when the service provided is part of a grant-funded program). An example of how cost can vary with consultation rate is shown in Figure 11.1. At high costs most forms of telehealth cannot compete against conventional ways of delivering health care, so the program soon becomes unsustainable in the commercial world. In this chapter we consider the choice of technology for a telehealth program as a major strategic investment. This investment must be grounded within the financial discipline of a business plan and must not be relegated to the status of an incidental capital investment decision or one individual's pursuit of a technological dream.

THE TELEHEALTH EQUIPMENT
INVESTMENT DECISION

It is frustrating when an organization spend tens or hundreds of thousands of dollars on telehealth equipment only to find 6 months later that the prices charged for the same hardware and software have dropped by as much as one third of what was originally charged. Progressive cost reductions are a fact of life when buying new information technology products, making the timing of any purchase of new equipment a critical decision. Investments in telehealth technology have to be made with the clear realization that they are inevitably associated with a considerable capital depreciation as the technology advances. Telehealth equipment must therefore generate sufficient revenue over its lifespan to cover this cost. Whether new equipment will reduce costs, increase business, or improve reliability of service is an important factor in the investment decision. Telehealth programs usually have to apportion overhead costs such as equipment purchase over the total number of consultations undertaken. If a telehealth program buys equipment that is too expensive for its purpose, low rates of consultation will result in unnecessarily high costs per consultation.

To compensate for rapid technological advancement telehealth programs are often advised to buy the highest-specification equipment their budgets can afford. Whether this is good advice depends on how realistically the equipment budget for the telehealth organization has been set. Ninety percent of telehealth programs are currently grant-funded, and most of these have based their equipment purchase decisions on spending the amount of grant money made available to them. This does not necessarily mean they have a sound business case for later selling commercial telehealth services. If a telehealth program expects to be a viable commercial venture, then it must cover its costs. Taking financial survival into consideration, a necessary caveat to add about equipment purchase is that a telehealth program

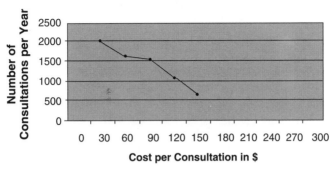

Figure 11.1 An illustrative example of the possible relationship between consultation rate and cost.

should purchase the highest-specification equipment available to meet its expected needs for delivering its core business activities at the lowest possible cost. This formula for purchasing telehealth equipment is shown in Figure 11.2.

The economic realities on which telehealth companies invest in telecommunications equipment should mirror similar investment processes in the telecommunications industry as a whole. Investment decisions in this industry are primarily based on knowledge about the expected number (rate) of calls and the volume of data (number of bytes) sent over time. In exactly the same way, any economic decisions about what telehealth equipment to buy must be based on the expected volume of usage of the system and the revenue this will generate. This commercial realism means that no rational economic justification exists for a telehealth organization spending four times more than necessary on equipment to develop a capacity to undertake teleradiology if it has not first identified a clear teleradiology market for it to exploit. Similarly, it makes no sense in an organization buying telehealth equipment requiring high-communications bandwidth to use its full functionality if this bandwidth is not going to be available. These situations are analogous to buying a car engineered to drive over 140 miles per hour when the speed limit on the roads is 70 miles per hour.

Figure 11.3 shows how any capital investment made by a commercial telehealth organization in communications equipment should be determined by the proportion of its projected revenue it can allocate to paying

Equipment purchased = Lowest cost for the functional applications required

Figure 11.2 A suggested formula for purchasing telehealth equipment.

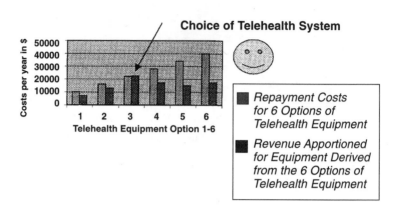

Figure 11.3   Choosing telehealth equipment.

for its purchase and running costs. If this revenue is insufficient to cover the costs of the equipment, the organization must either rethink its business plan or reconsider whether it should be in the business of telehealth at all.

The Purchase of Telehealth Equipment

Several important practical decisions associated with purchasing telehealth equipment are shown in Table 11.1. Telehealth equipment does not necessarily have to be specifically designed for use in telehealth. Standard "off the shelf" videoconferencing equipment can sometimes serve the same function. Off-the-shelf technology is often cheaper, easier to support, and available to buy at short notice. Its disadvantages:

1. The range of peripheral equipment needed, ranging from microscopes to stethoscopes, may either not be available or need considerable adaptation to work on the system.
2. Equipment that is not made for medical purposes may not meet the necessary quality standards for health care use.

Before buying telehealth systems it is important to weigh the benefits of outright purchase against lease of the equipment. This calculation often shows that the eventual costs of leasing are higher in the long term than an outright purchase. The seeming price advantage of purchasing equipment can be offset by the way the organization intending to operate the telehealth

Table 11.1   Purchasing Considerations for Telehealth Equipment

- Whether to buy bespoke telehealth equipment or purchase off-the-shelf computer and telecommunications equipment
- Whether to purchase the equipment outright or to lease it
- Arrangements for warranty and support
- Whether to adopt an open systems approach or a closed system approach to the systems design

system accounts for the capital charges of any new equipment purchases. Capital charges relating to equipment purchase over a certain limit may be costs a telehealth program must add to the price it charges for its services. This additional cost may affect the competitiveness of the service and so make leasing the preferred method of equipment acquisition instead of purchase.

For a telehealth service to effectively replace conventional face-to-face methods of delivering health care, adequate arrangements must be in place in case of a system failure. The type of service to be provided is what determines the exact requirements for systems backup and support. Backup arrangements an operational telehealth service may need to consider are suggested by Table 11.2 and Figures 11.4 to 11.6.

The equipment purchased for a telehealth system may need to fit with either an open systems approach or a closed systems approach. An open systems approach is one where the network architecture, the hardware configuration, and the software configuration are open and compatible with other systems. This approach offers a flexible system that is easy to use and can communicate with other users. A closed system is one in which a supplier, whether of the network, the hardware, or the software, offers a product that binds the purchaser into a system where access to other technology and other users may be difficult. Because of the huge national and international market for telehealth and the number of different systems already operating to provide telehealth services, a rule in purchasing telehealth equipment

Table 11.2   Backup in Case of Telehealth Equipment Failure

- Access to a dial-up diagnostic service that offers immediate assessment of the problem and enables maintenance engineers to reconfigure software faults remotely
- A 24-hour on-site repair service to assess and correct any equipment faults if the remote diagnostics cannot remedy the problem
- An equipment replacement option to get the service operational if on-site repair of the fault is not possible

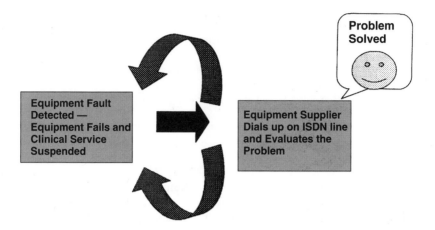

Figure 11.4   Remote diagnosis of a telehealth equipment failure.

should be to look for open-systems architecture whenever possible. The reason for not using closed-systems architecture is highlighted in Table 11.3.

The Vendor

The choice of a vendor for telehealth equipment is crucial, and it involves thinking about more than just the price and equipment specification. Unfortunately, many telehealth equipment suppliers and telecommunications companies have viewed telehealth as a new market where they as vendors are in the business of selling as much equipment and as much bandwidth to their customers as possible. Their interest is in "selling boxes," and the only limit on their sales is what the customer can eventually pay. Although this approach of maximizing sales is an entirely natural one in a commercial environment, it is also shortsighted because it does not nurture the long-term market for telehealth products. It is as unwise to automatically consider that a telehealth equipment supplier will offer good advice on what equipment to buy as it is in any other area of commerce.

Price and specification are important when buying telehealth equipment, but so also is ensuring that equipment from different manufacturers is compatible and ensuring that any service agreements for the supply and maintenance of equipment are clear and unambiguous. For example, if a newly purchased teledermatology camera does not transmit pictures, is it a problem with the camera or with a software interface on the computer? Responsibilities for the functioning and compatibility of any equipment provided must be clearly assigned. It is an unpleasant and avoidable headache if these areas of technical responsibility have to be resolved at a

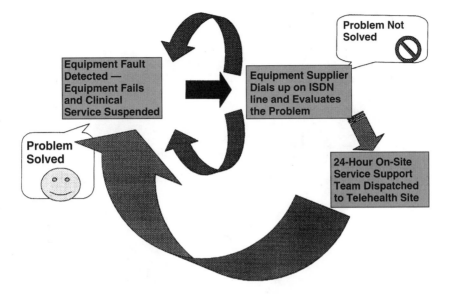

Figure 11.5   On-site telehealth equipment maintenance.

time when delays in offering services lose vital credibility and revenue for a telehealth program. Lack of clarity about responsibilities for equipment warranty immediately put a telehealth program in a weak negotiating position. It is wise to choose a telehealth equipment manufacturer who can supply and support a wide range of equipment and who will provide overall responsibility for sorting out problems if anything goes wrong. This is invariably a supplier who is interested in the development of telehealth and not just in making short-term profits from the sale of boxes.

HOW DATA EXCHANGE PERFORMANCE RATES DETERMINE THE OPERATIONAL FUTURE OF COMMERCIAL TELEHEALTH PROGRAMS

Commercial telehealth companies are in the business of offering remote health care transactions. If the health care products (e.g., dermatology

Table 11.3   Problems with Closed System Architecture

Choosing closed system architecture for a telehealth system imposes limitations on the flexibility and connectivity of the service. This means that access to the growing market opportunities for telehealth may be unnecessarily limited because of incompatibilities between networks, software, and hardware.

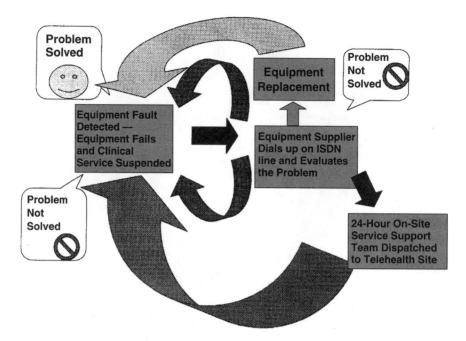

Figure 11.6   Telehealth equipment exchange.

consultation, remote x-ray interpretation, or remote diagnostic pathology report) are in demand, then the efficiency, quality, and cost of the data exchange process may be what decide whether providing telehealth services is a viable commercial proposition.

Efficiency of Data Transmission

Organizations wanting to purchase telehealth services define the technical efficiency of the systems they want in relatively simple terms. They expect a service to work when and where they demand it and to complete the processes of data exchange within a required operational timescale.

Quality of Data Transmission

The quality of data transmission demanded by customers who purchase telehealth services is viewed by them simply as a having data/images transmitted clearly enough for the purpose required and reliably enough that there is no need to retransmit the data.

Cost of Data Transmission

Depending on the geographical locations for a telehealth service, the costs of data transmission, including the line installation, line rental charges, and call charges (or the lease of the line), may amount to as much as 15% to 25% of the total cost of providing the telehealth service (however, these costs are continually falling). This makes one of the jobs for a telehealth provider organization to find ways to titrate these costs against the quality and efficiency requirements for data transfer, the objective being to offer a competitive telehealth service specification that health care providers can afford to buy. Currently, a range of data exchange media are available for a telehealth system to use for telehealth transactions; these are shown in Table 11.4.

Differences in the efficiency, quality, and cost benefits of each of these four data transmission media mean that practical considerations define which is best to use in a particular situation. A POTS (plain old telephone system) data transmission may be appropriate for transmitting low volumes of nonurgent x-rays between two destinations for a teleradiology service. A high volume of x-rays and a need for urgent reporting may necessitate an ISDN (integrated services digital network) or T1 connection in another teleradiology situation. In practical terms the current convention used to specify the data transmission needs of telehealth systems is defined in terms of the bandwidth requirement. Bandwidth measures the capacity of the transmission medium (carrier) to transmit data (bits) over time (seconds). The formula for this is shown in Figure 11.7.

If the bandwidth connects users between two points, it is termed a point-to-point telehealth service. If the bandwidth connection links multiple points, it is then a telehealth network. The design of any telehealth system, whether point to point or networked, must decide how it will be connected onto a digital data system. Most health care providers that are seriously interested in adopting telehealth often have their own local area network (LAN, defined as when the terminal distance from the server is less than 1 kilometer) in place to distribute information. If so, an emerging issue for them is explore whether they can provide telehealth services on their own LAN or use the LAN as the portal of access onto a wide area network (WAN, defined as when the terminal distance from the server is greater than 1 kilometer) or a switched network. The significance of these decisions relates to data networking of clinicians and the strategic implications of whether a telehealth service can interface with an integrated patient record. Making these links often poses dilemmas for systems design and conflicts about using open systems and their data security in relation to confidential patient information.

$$\text{Bandwidth (kilobits/second)} = \frac{\text{Amount of data transmitted}}{\text{Unit time}}$$

Figure 11.7   The definition of bandwidth.

Table 11.4   Data Exchange Media for Telehealth

Type of data exchange medium	Example
Copper wire	POTS (plain old telephone service)
Optical fiber	ISDN/cable TV systems
Radio	Cellular telephone systems
Microwave	Satellite transmission systems

BUYING BANDWIDTH

How to network data is yet another crucial technical decision for a telehealth system. Currently, this is because obtaining bandwidth and getting it at the right price are important operational and financial considerations for any telehealth system. In the future this is likely to become much less important. A long-term vision preoccupying the boardrooms of many telecommunications companies is how they will deal with a future scenario in which virtually unlimited bandwidth is available on demand at virtually no cost. In this scenario the future business of telecommunications companies may switch away from supplying bandwidth to participating in the supply of value-added services on their network (e.g., Internet services and telehealth). In this case they will no longer be simple carriers of information. Whether they remain as simple data carriers or become suppliers of value-added services, telecommunications companies often place their own interests first (as most industries do) when it comes to selling bandwidth. This is yet another reason to adopt an open systems approach to networking in telehealth. In the short term an open systems strategy means that a telehealth provider can shop around for bandwidth at competitive rates, and in the longer term it does not face having its route to market strictly controlled. Becoming reliant on a closed network may place a telehealth system in an unnecessarily vulnerable situation in the future.

The freedom of telehealth systems to choose their carrier is often determined geographically. In metropolitan areas telehealth systems may have a choice of carrier, including traditional telecommunications suppliers and new entrants to the market such as cable TV companies. In rural areas the choice of carrier may be limited to a single provider.

The short-term interest of telecommunications companies is in getting the highest revenue they can from selling their current bandwidth capacity. In the United States this has resulted in many telehealth services being provided on leased data lines that are expensive. The telecom industry would still make money on leased T1 lines if they charged $2 per mile per month rather than the $16 per mile per month some currently charge.[192] For tele-health programs generating low volumes of telehealth transactions, developing a WAN using leased data lines may not be a cost-effective way of buying bandwidth. Telehealth programs must look at the traditional options of using a LAN, a WAN, or a dial-up switched network to deliver services, as well as new Internet-associated options (e.g., Intranets and Extranets). Which option a telehealth program chooses will depend on factors such as those shown in Table 11.5.

In the United Kingdom a practical concern for health care organizations interested in telehealth is whether or not to use the dedicated WAN for the National Health Service, the NHS Wide Network. The issues connected with data security favor this closed system, whereas the future growth of the Internet and cost considerations may favor an open systems approach with due attention to data security. The area of supplying data network services is dynamically changing. It is not possible to provide a simple formula to help telehealth programs to decide what option to chose. Some comparisons between current choices are shown in Table 11.6. For practical reasons many telehealth systems opt to provide telehealth services using the switched net-work or leased lines of a major telecommunications carrier and rarely use a packet network such as a LAN. The reasons for this are shown in Table 11.7.

A telehealth program can purchase bandwidth by leasing lines or by paying rental and call charges. The relative benefit of each method of purchasing bandwidth depends on the volume of telehealth transactions occurring. Although sophisticated telehealth activity such as teleradiology can take place using analog data systems such as a POTS working at 33 Kbps (kilobits per second) with compression, most telehealth activity uses digital data systems (DDS). The common choices available for DDS are switched-56, DS0, ISDN, ATM, or satellite.

Switched-56

The most familiar DDS available to most consumers is that provided at 56 kbps on the POTS (plain old telephone system) and this is called switched-56. This service is available at most geographic locations. If a telehealth service uses switched-56, users can simply dial up to get the required services. Monitoring of telehealth activity and billing for the costs of the digital data transfer can be arranged in conjunction with the telecommunications company providing the switched-56 service. To deliver switched-56 services within a 2-mile radius of their local exchange a telecommunications company can use a single pair of copper wires. Once the distance is above 2 miles it requires two pairs of wires, and depending on the exact distance, it also

Table 11.5   Factors to Consider in Buying Network Capacity

- Capital and revenue costs of each option
- The amount of bandwidth required by the telehealth applications
- The number of calls of calls per month
- Data security
- The number of system users
- The geographical distribution of the users
- The reliability of the service

may mean amplifying the signal with a repeater. The need for amplification also depends on whether wire, cable, or optical fiber is the available transmission medium. The practical significance of the need to modify cable or amplify the signal is that it can result in delays for telehealth providers in obtaining a connection and can increase costs.

DS Zero (DS0)

This service option provides data transmission at a rate of 64 Kbps. As with switched-56, data transmission is initiated by direct dialing. The physical management of this data exchange works through a proportion of the 64 Kbps allocated for switching and signaling purposes. This "in-band" requirement of 8 Kbps used for data management allows a dedicated circuit to be set up between two points, for example, a telehealth remote site and the hub site. The amount of bandwidth required is the same as providing digital-quality telephone services. Individual channels of DS0 can be aggregated together by multiplexing to offer larger amounts of bandwidth. These are in multiples of 64 Kbps that are provided as shown in Figure 11.8.

Integrated Services Digital Network

This is a communications protocol for the transmission of digital data to communicate integrated audio, video, and data signals to homes and businesses. Integrated services digital network (ISDN) solves the problem of how to use a variety of inherited cabling options to cover the final distances from telecom exchanges up to buildings. It allows high bandwidth to be brought into the office and the home without expensive investment in rewiring. ISDN is widely available in the United Kingdom but less so in the United States. The advantage of ISDN to telehealth providers is that they can use a partnership or commercial arrangement with a telecommunications company to offer a digital network facility to health care organizations at relatively low cost. In practice the delays in installation and operation of ISDN can be frustrating, and it can be an expensive option if the usage

Table 11.6   Features of Different Types of Network for Telehealth

Type of network	Features	Broad advantages	Broad disadvantages
Local area network (LAN)	Closed network within a kilometer of the server, usually a packet network	Suits an organization confined to a small geographical area that has a need to keep control of its data systems.	There are problems with data security on a LAN unless there are enforced protocols for the users and the locations that have access.
Wide area network (WAN)	Dedicated private circuit using leased lines, switched lines such as ISDN, X.25, or frame relay	Provides a cost-effective means of exchanging data between distant sites for messaging and telehealth.	The costs of the WAN may be high, particularly if leased lines are used.
Switched network	A dial-up access to bandwidth using DS zero, ISDN, or ATM	Offers the possibility of bandwidth on demand that is cheaper and more flexible. It is also easier to use if offering telehealth services to distant locations.	The availability of switched networked services is patchy, especially in rural areas. They are still expensive. There are often delays in installation.
Intranet	A private Internet linked to the public Internet through tightly controlled data gateways	This uses the same TCP/IP protocols as are used on the Internet. It can also use the Web browsers and applications languages such as JAVA.	There is the need for data security through developing firewalls that must be maintained to protect data confidentiality.
Extranet	This is an area that is created between the two routers that separate the public Internet from an Intranet.	Provides data sources that can be accessed by the public Internet and also by Intranet/s. This can make information processing and distribution more efficient.	The contents of these databases are currently complex to maintain. In large organizations rigorous management is needed and. data security is an important consideration.

Table 11.7   Benefits of a Switched Network to a Telehealth Provider

- A switched network is a flexible way of providing services to two or more users who are remote from each other.
- Other users can be added relatively easily.
- Switched networks are more secure.
- Data transmission on packet networks is more prone to error and to suffer delay in transmission.

volume is high. ISDN is available at similar multiples of bandwidth to DS0, from 128 Kbps upward. ISDN is a convenient and flexible way of providing telehealth services requiring two-way interactive video. Again, as with DS0, ISDN is available through direct dialing. This makes it flexible and convenient to use. It also means billing for telecommunications services can be negotiated directly with the telecommunications company.

Asynchronous Transfer Mode

Another data transfer protocol available for transmitting digital data, this commercial service can be purchased from telecommunications companies that offer bandwidth on demand. Data, video, and audio needs of telehealth transactions can be served by one line, and the demand for varying data transmission rates is met by dynamically reallocating bandwidth as and when it is needed. In telehealth this is typically useful when there is a variable requirement for high bandwidths to communicate real-time audio and video information over long distances to health care sites separated by large geographical distances. The supply of this bandwidth capacity depends on the availability of high-capacity fiberoptic cabling systems such as OC-3 and OC-12. These channels are expensive and not readily available in rural areas, so the choice of asynchronous transfer mode (ATM) depends on a judgment of the variability in the volumes of data transfer taking place and the relative concentration of the services provided in rural versus metropolitan areas. ATM is a flexible dial-up service billed through the telecommunications carrier. When permanent virtual circuits (PVCs) are used with ATM, these offer many of the advantages of leased lines at much lower costs. An option instead of ATM now being offered by some telecommunication providers is frame relay, a packet network service that is now able to work at OC3 speeds.

Satellite vs. Wired Bandwidth for Telehealth

There is great potential to provide telehealth services in Asia and Africa, where the cost of providing specialist medical expertise based on the traditional

- **64 Kbps**   **DS zero**
- **128 Kbps**   **X 2 DS zero**
- **384 Kbps**   **X 6 DS zero**
- **768 Kbps**   **x12 DS zero**

Figure 11.8   Multiples of 64 Kbps service provision.

hospital is often prohibitively expensive. A medical problem that a generalist doctor might see on average once every 15 years is handled less well than a problem she/he sees 10 times a week. Telehealth offers a way to bring the specialist to the patient in cost-effective ways in developing countries unable to afford this type of medical care. Although this potential market for telehealth exists in developing countries, data transmission problems currently prohibit its routine use. Digital data connections do not exist, and the data transmission costs by satellite are currently too high to make this a practicable proposition in most instances. We have had some experience of trying to develop the business case for telehealth services to support spinal injuries care and infectious disease diagnosis and care in developing countries. When the costs of transmitting data from real-time videoconsultation and x-rays falls, these services will be cost-effective in terms of improved patient outcomes.

If the predicted global satellite data networks are able to offer low-cost telecommunications facilities to developing countries, this will open up exciting new prospects in providing medical care. To be useful for telehealth applications these must be satellites in low earth orbit, and the cost of the transmitting stations must drop. Currently, the signal delay and the cost of the transmitting equipment make telehealth nonviable in overseas situations where the medical, nursing, physical therapy, and occupational therapy needs are high, and telehealth could benefit the delivery of health care to the general population.

Choosing How to Buy Bandwidth

The advantage of buying bandwidth in the form of ISDN or ATM from a telecommunications company as opposed to setting up a dedicated network for a telehealth system depends on the geographical spread of the service and the volume of data transfer. Dial-up bandwidth is billed on the simple formula shown in Figure 11.9.

The technology now available for telehealth offers exciting new visions of how health care will be provided in the future. Despite the reduction in the costs of telehealth equipment and bandwidth, these are often still too high to develop a doable business case for a telehealth application. Many people

Cost ∝ (time of call) and (distance apart of parties involved in call)

Figure 11.9   Typical formula for the billing of bandwidth.

are purists about telehealth and how it should be defined. One practical consequence of this is to make telehealth programs reluctant to see telehealth in a wider perspective. If high bandwidth costs and low levels of usage are significant financial barriers to the viability of a telehealth service, then creative solutions often exist in forming collaborations with other possible users of the technology. A critical mass of applications may be needed to make a telehealth network workable. A telehealth provider can form alliances with other organizations to deliver

- Distance education and training of health care professionals
- Information to schools and libraries in rural areas
- Data with commercial or industrial organizations as partners in the network

EQUIPMENT AND COMMUNICATION STANDARDS

A major reason for the failure and obsolescence of computing and telecommunications equipment is incompatible technical standards.

Videoconferencing Standards

Telehealth programs can use off-the-shelf or proprietary technology for videoconferencing. This may be fine when the service provided is limited to a small group of users, all of whom use the same equipment. It becomes a problem when the service wants to link to other users or there is a need to upgrade the equipment and consider other manufacturers. Incompatibility of equipment can then became a problem and make it unnecessarily expensive to stay in the business of teleconsultation. There are now videoconferencing standards for transmission over POTS—H.324, ISDN, and switched-circuit H.320 and Ethernet H.323. There are also standards under development for bridging among H.323, H.324, and H.320. These bridging standards are vital to consider in the design of the systems architecture for a telehealth program and should help resolve the problem of incompatibility among various systems. Health care providers who have their physicians' offices on an Ethernet network are looking at ways of linking into a switched network and making the process of teleconsultation cheaper and more convenient.

Digital Imaging Standards

The American College of Radiology and the National Electrical Manufacturers Association have developed the Digital Image Communication in Medicine (DICOM) standard[193]—the ACR-NEMA Version 3 (DICOM). This standard began as a way of harmonizing the hardware and software used to display images from digital imaging equipment such as CT scanners. The standard applies to the networking of digital information as applied to a picture archiving and communication system (PACS). It does not yet apply to how data is transferred on a teleradiology system. If a DICOM standard is adopted for the transmission of teleradiology data, it gives the system versatility of use and compatibility. The DICOM standard is currently under review to see how applicable it may be to the transmission of digital data from other specialties such as cardiology, pathology and nuclear medicine.

Data Compression Standards

A codec is a device that codes and then decodes video information. A codec reduces the amount of data transmission required over a telehealth network to send and receive full-motion video. This data reduction is achieved by removing redundant or superfluous information from the video signal and simplifying the process of data exchange. The amount of redundant and superfluous information present is inversely proportional to the amount of movement taking place and the fine detail in the images captured by the videocamera. A variety of industry standards of codec exist, and the choice of codec for a telehealth program depends on the exact clinical requirement. Real-time fetal ultrasound scanning to detect intrauterine abnormalities requires more bandwidth and a more expensive codec than a face-to-face videoconsultation involving "talking heads." Codecs can be synchronous or asynchronous. Asynchronous means that the video signal is decoded more easily than it is encoded. The emerging new standard is MPEG2, an asynchronous codec technology. Unfortunately, the high cost of the encoder can make this uneconomic for two-way videoconsultation. It is important when procuring a telehealth system for videoconferencing to consider the codec technology because of the cost implications this will have for high-resolution clinical applications.

Audio Quality in Telehealth Applications

The quality of the audio transmission is often taken for granted when drawing up telehealth equipment specifications. Usually, far more thought is given to the video reproduction. When real-time videoconferencing systems are used in clinical situations, poor audio quality and the discomfort this causes can be a reason why patients and physicians reject using telehealth. Demonstrations of telehealth equipment can be misleading about the audio quality of an operational system, particularly when both the remote and hub ends of the equipment are demonstrated in the same building by the manufacturer. The independent or compounded result of poor acoustics in the teleconsultation suite, transmission delay, and the effects of separate audio channels can result in intolerable echo distortions of the sound reproduction for the patient and practitioner. Poor audio is often a reason that patients, especially when they are elderly, prefer face-to-face consultations instead of telehealth. Resolving these problems by attention to this detail at the time of equipment purchase is easier than doing so when the system is in place.

In addition to the effect of audio quality on the spoken voice, the quality of audio transmission has an effect on the diagnosis of chest and heart disease using a remote stethoscope. Just as the reproduction of a Mozart symphony is affected by the quality of the sound equipment and its frequency response, so too are cardiac and chest auscultation. If the diagnosis of chest and heart disease is a component of the telehealth service being offered, then sufficient attention must be paid to the audio quality in the equipment specification.

EQUIPMENT REQUIREMENTS FOR SPECIFIC TELEHEALTH APPLICATIONS

General Points on Choosing Equipment for Clinical Applications

The purchase of telehealth equipment should be with a clear specification in mind for each element to be purchased, guided by the clinical needs of the service and the budget available to buy equipment. The practitioners who will use the equipment must be involved in the decision about what to purchase. The practitioners' choice of system specification must be based on sound reasoning and evidence to support the functionality they demand from each element of the specification. There is rarely one standard system for all clinical situations. For example, the requirements for a teledermatology service may range from a simple personal computer–based store-and-forward system to a real-time videoconferencing system costing much more and requiring more bandwidth. The choice of which to buy must be based on the demands of providing a clinical service appropriately. It is important to make objective decisions about equipment purchase. Spending more on equipment than necessary to please a clinician or manager who is enamored of a shiny new toy is a mistake. It is equally a mistake to insist on keeping absolutely to an agreed-to budget if the equipment will not meet the clinical requirements of delivering the service. It is then much better to renegotiate the budget. Elements to include in the equipment purchase for a telehealth application are shown in Table 11.8.

Teleradiology System Specification

Digital Image Capture Systems

The x-ray image capture in a teleradiology system can take place either by direct digitization of the x-ray image at the time of the x-ray exposure, or by digitizing an x-ray film taken on a conventional x-ray system using a scanner. Direct digitization of the x-ray can obviate the need for x-ray film and for x-ray processing equipment. The resulting x-ray image can be stored temporarily on a computer hard drive and then archived on a device such as an optical disk, or it can be immediately distributed and stored on a network (e.g., a PACS). A less expensive solution in terms of capital cost is to use a scanner to digitize the normal images taken for x-ray, CT, and MRI and send them for remote reporting. Direct digitization and "high end" scanners can produce diagnostic quality images (ACR-NEMA standard of at least 2Kx2Kx12-bit capture.

Lower-tech solutions that produce interim/preliminary read-quality images are to transmit the x-ray using a cheaper "low end" scanner or place the x-ray on an x-ray screen and capture the image using a videocamera.

Digital Data Transmission Systems

Once the digital image has been taken, it must be tagged and labeled with the patient's details before it can be stored or moved around. This can be accomplished on a network by interfacing the digital image to a microcomputer and distributing it on a LAN. Using the DICOM standard the digital images can be distributed and stored on a PACS. Finally, using DICOM standards or proprietary compression techniques, the digital images can be sent over digital data networks to other sites for reporting. The digital data system can be DS0, ISDN, or ATM, depending on the availability, cost, and urgency of reporting required.

Digital Data Receiver and Display Systems

After its transmission, digital teleradiology data must be decoded. If diagnostic-quality images are required for reporting, they must be viewed on special radiographic digital display monitors. The quality of the images produced by videomonitors for teleradiology have been a source of contention

Table 11.8   Elements to Consider in the Specification of a Telehealth System

- Digital image capture system
- Digital data transmission system
- Digital data connection
- Digital data receiver system
- Digital data display system
- Storage and archive system
- Patient information system interface

because of concerns whether they can match the image resolution of the x-ray film. This lack of resolution is not because of the pixel content of the display, typically 2000 pixels × 2000 lines. The problem is with the level of contrast available—usually less than 100 shades of grayscale. This deficiency can be compensated for by special techniques such as

- Histogram-based image transformation
- Filter-based image transformation
- Unsharp mask

These techniques give a radiologist the ability to use "window" and "level" control to manipulate the images and get adequate contrast distinction for confident reporting.

Storage and Archive Systems and the Patient Information System Interface

Serious commercial teleradiology means that labeling information, distributing x-ray images, and sending reports are automated processes. Many grant-funded teleradiology projects and small-scale commercial teleradiology operations can obviate the capital investment and complexity of organizing these processes by digitizing x-ray films and by sending word-processed reports via a fax machine. Serious commercial teleradiology services solve these by linking to a PACS or using a proprietary indexing and archiving system. Automating these processes can be a major problem when trying to scale up the activity of a small teleradiology operation. Web-based digital storage and display are a recent advance enabling clinicians to view images at remote locations.

Store-and-Forward Teledermatology System Specification

Digital Image Capture System

The digital data capture system in teledermatology is a digital camera that takes still images. A wide range of digital cameras is available off the shelf for use in teledermatology. Additional specialized diagnostic devices are available, including

- Episcopes that give 22x magnification of the epidermis
- Polarizing dermatology microscopes that give 10–1000x magnification
- Dermatoscopes

Many of these devices come with lighting systems designed to complement the system and help with color resolution.

Digital Data Transmission Systems and Patient Information Systems Interface

The advantage of the store-and-forward system is that clinicians can report diagnostic images at their convenience. These diagnostic images may include still images and video clips. For medicolegal purposes and good housekeeping of the images (e.g., teledermatology images) a patient identifier and clinical history must be combined with the images before they are stored or sent for reporting. Although a variety of nonspecialist commercial software packages can be adapted to use for store-and-forward teledermatology, custom-made solutions are available. These solutions bundle patient demographic data, patient records, and photographic images (including x-rays) into a multimedia patient record that can be sent to the reporting consultant, such as a dermatologist.

Digital Data Connection, Digital Data Receiving and Display

Store-and-forward teledermatology images can be sent on a range of data links; these include a LAN, a WAN, POTS, ISDN, ATM. The data content is usually modest, and there is less clinical urgency, so the least expensive option should be chosen. Because of data security concerns the Internet has not been a currently favored method of data transmission. The most common method of receiving information and displaying the images is a personal computer. However, advances in encription make Web solutions an option now.

A Real-Time Video Teleconsultation System Specification

Digital Image Capture System

The digital data capture system used in a teleconsultation system (e.g., teledermatology) is a digital videocamera. This takes real-time images of the patient and enables a consulting specialist (e.g., a dermatologist) to directly take a history from the patient. The adequacy of the camera resolution and the color verisimilitude are important determinants of whether an accurate diagnosis is made. Therefore, the choice of camera equipment and its specification should rest with the dermatologists reporting the teledermatology cases. A wide range of digital videocameras that can be used for teledermatology are available off the shelf. The general specification of these for interactive teledermatology usually includes the following specifications:

- 1–50x zoom capacity
- Push-button polarization to reduce skin reflection
- Auto focus and auto white balance
- Composite or S-video output
- Built-in freeze-frame capacity

The lighting of the patient is particularly important, and many systems come with integrated light and video to avoid the cumbersome problem of moving a lamp while examining a patient. As with store-and-forward dermatology, optional specialized diagnostic devices are available in teledermatology:

- Videoepiscopes that give 22x magnification of the epidermis
- Videodermatoscopes

Like the still-image devices, these usually come with lighting systems designed to complement the system and help with color resolution. Some controversy exists about the value these systems add to teledermatology.

Digital Data Transmission Systems and Patient Information Systems Interface

The video camera links to a codec to transmit the digital data. This allows an interactive patient consultation to take place and the history, findings on remote examination, and images of the patient to be viewed directly by a remote specialist (e.g., a dermatologist). It is not yet mandatory for any specific patient data to be exchanged or for the teleconsultation system to interface with the patient information system.

Digital Data Connection, Digital Data Receiving and Display

ISDN2 is usually the lowest requirement for realistic interactive videoconferencing (e.g., for teledermatology). Most videocameras have a freeze-frame capability to send more detailed still images when required. It usually helps to fix the camera on a tripod when doing this to get the best possible quality image; otherwise, movement artifact can still be a problem. The most common method of receiving information and displaying the images is either on a modified personal computer or on a dedicated videoconferencing system.

Telepathology System Specifications

Telepathology systems are usually store-and-forward or real-time interactive systems. They therefore face many of the same technical issues as apply to teledermatology. The main reasons to choose a real-time interactive telepathology system instead of a store-and-forward system are

1. If a relatively small amount of data is sent
2. If interactive reporting must take place

If the pathology technician or pathologist at the remote end and the specialist at the reporting end can both view the specimen under low magnification and then increase the magnification when an area of abnormality is detected, this simulates the usual diagnostic pathology examination. When diagnostic pathology slides are reported conventionally, the pathologist switches between low- and high-resolution objectives on the microscope to focus on any abnormalities.

A real-time interactive diagnostic pathology examination can take place with a camera attachment to a microscope. This can be frustrating and cumbersome for the reporting pathologist. For this reason many pathologists prefer to use a videomicroscope with a remotely movable carriage and identify directly areas of abnormality themselves.

The issues of linkage of the images in store-and-forward to a multimedia patient record apply to telepathology as they do to teleradiology and teledermatology.

Telepsychiatry, Teleophthalmology, Remote Emergency Medical Care, Telecardiology, and Teleorthopedics

These branches of health care use interactive videoconferencing, and the technical issues they raise are essentially the same as ones already covered in teledermatology. There is a wide range of accessories, some examples of which are listed below to extend the capacity of these applications.

Tele–Home Care

Some of the remote monitoring devices available for home care are listed in Table 11.9. The main technical problems that telehealth programs face

Table 11.9   Examples of Add-On Devices to Extend the Scope of Telehealth

Cardiology
- Digital stethoscopes
- Twelve-lead ECG
- Echocardiograph transmission

Remote pacemaker monitoring
- Dentistry
- Dental cameras

Home monitoring
- Transtelephonic ECG
- Remote spirometry FVC, FEV_1, FEV_{50}
- Peak flow monitoring
- Pulse oximetry
- Temperature monitoring
- Monitoring of infusion pumps
- Remote blood pressure monitoring

Neurology
- Transtelephonic electroencephalograms

Ophthalmology
- Video ophthalmoscopes
- Video slit lamps
- Video funduscopes

Orthopedics
- Remote arthroscopy

Otolaryngology
- Fiberoptic otoscopes
- Videonasopharyngoscopes
- Throat illuminators
- Videolaryngoscopes

Surgery
- Remote laparoscopy
- Remote endoscopy

when they monitor patients at home instead of in a hospital is a much wider variation in the data captured than is typically expected in hospital care. Setting the correct thresholds for intervention is a major initial challenge for home monitoring programs because a frequent justification for these programs is to save the costs of hospital care. If the thresholds for intervention are set incorrectly for patients, then unnecessary and costly hospital admissions and home visits can occur instead of reducing admissions.

Consumer Telehealth Devices

A rapidly emerging area of telehealth is the marriage between the medical device industry and the Internet. A plethora of medical devices from heart monitors to infusion pumps can now be intelligently coupled to expert systems via the Web. Some of these devices very clearly have their ownership and application within the traditional world of health care and health care practice. However, new technologies are about to emerge that bring this sophistication to the ordinary consumer in the home. Medical devices are under beta testing in areas such as gynecology to remotely monitor body temperature. These devices have applications for managing contraception by the rhythm method and determining optimal fertility, thereby helping to decide the optimal time to engage in or restrain from sexual intercourse. Future develpments in this technology hold promise to help in managing incontinence in women.

12

Other Important Influences on Health Care That Affect the Future of Telehealth

Both countries and individuals invest in purchasing health care services because they want to improve levels of health and guard against the effects of ill health. Until the late 1980s, governments believed a simple mantra that suggested that if they simply spent more money on health care they would improve their population's health. This approach sounds naïve now. If telehealth technology had been as technically sophisticated in the 1980s as it is now and had cost less, it could well have been widely introduced with little questioning. This would have been possible then, solely based on the promise that telehealth could improve people's health without needing to provide actual evidence that it did so. CT and MRI imaging are examples of technologies that were accepted relatively unquestioningly then. Times change, and now telehealth has to earn its place in a world where a very different environment exists for deciding how to incorporate new health care technologies into practice.

Government, health insurers, and many individual patients now readily dismiss the idea of a directly proportional relationship between what is spent on health care services and any improvements in health that result, as suggested in Figure 12.1. This change in attitude of government and health insurers toward health care spending is not associated with a particular nihilism about the use of health care interventions. Instead, it places an

Health Care Expenditure α Improved Health

Figure 12.1   Health ≈ health care spending—a discredited equation.

onus on anybody introducing new health care interventions to prove that they improve health and are cost-effective. Improved health and cost-effectiveness are therefore positive outcomes expected of any new health care intervention. Outcomes measurement provides a way of analyzing the effects of a new health care intervention such as telehealth and communicating these data to health care purchasers so they can consider using it. Merely demonstrating that positive outcomes are associated with a new health care intervention is not usually sufficient to make a case for health care purchasers to adopt it. It also must be quite clear that the process of care was applied consistently and the outcomes measured were directly attributable to this process of care. Clinical standard setting and clinical audit can make this causal connection and link clinical processes to clinical outcomes. Taken together, outcome measurement, clinical audit, and clinical standard setting are ways of providing evidence that health care interventions are appropriate, clinically effective, and cost-effective, that is, that there is "evidence" for using them in practice.

In this chapter we look at some important processes that telehealth programs need to understand because they help to show that health care interventions are evidence-based. Similar tools and techniques are used for clinical audit and outcomes measurement and can be useful to a telehealth program for clinical risk management and new product development. Unfortunately many clinicians and managers in health care still fail to see the writing on the wall, that ongoing assessment and evaluation of the services they provide is now an essential requirement, not an optional extra to delivering care. It is no longer good enough to express an opinion about the need to provide a particular health care intervention unless this is backed up by evidence. Telehealth programs have everything to gain and very little to lose by being proactive in offering evidence to prove that telehealth is both clinically effective and cost-effective to health care purchasers. These help in developing a sound business case and at the same time benefit patients.

OUTCOMES MEASUREMENT

Until recently, it was largely taken for granted that the health of an individual or a population was improved by providing health care services. Health care services were usually seen as synonymous with employing health care professionals (e.g., doctors and nurses) to provide care in whatever way they thought best. If government officials wanted to show they had improved health care, they quoted statistics to show how many more doctors and nurses were employed during their term of office. This created a self-perpetuating system. Doctors and nurses existed to improve health and "do good"; therefore, employing doctors and nurses must de facto "do good" and improve health. The solution to any health care problem became simply employing more health care professionals. The management of those resources was not an issue.

A combination of events has changed this situation. The major precipitants of this change were the inflationary effects of new technology in health care and of an aging population demanding ever more health care services. Expenditure on health care is threatening to gobble up more and more of countries' gross domestic product. Inevitably, a time had to arrive when questions were asked about what tangible benefits to health resulted from this investment. Wide variations were found in how individual clinicians practiced, showing how similar patients in different geographical areas could receive different treatments based on the preference of the clinician and not on the condition of the patient.[53] It was impossible to tell whether the health of men in one state, where prostate surgery rates were twice those in another state, had better health as a result. There were no outcome measures. Once research moved from looking at the process of care to the outcome of care, it became clear that only 20% of current health care practice is based on any clear evidence of its effectiveness.[194] This is not to say that the other 80% of health care is not effective, just that we do not know whether it is or not.

As concerned health care purchasers facing escalating health care costs, government and health insurers are making the natural leap to specifying the purchase of services with proven good outcomes. Health care systems have grown like Topsy. Because of cost inflation the future purchasing of health care services is unlikely to be based on buying more of the same. When it is suggested that patients are going to benefit from an intervention or to suffer without it, purchasers of health care want to see the evidence on which these assertions are based. They want to see data showing the outcomes of an intervention for patients as well as hearing the opinion of clinicians. Many clinicians still find it difficult to accept that health care should be based on objective evidence for the treatments they give benefiting patients. Clinicians often make the following kinds of statements: "I know what my patients want" and "Facts, what facts? I know that this treatment works." It is not within the scope of this book to debate the rights and wrongs of this position, only to point out the way external circumstances are altering. We see outcomes measurement as an inevitable part of how health care will be practiced in the future. If telehealth is to be a tool with any role to play in the practice of health care in this future, it must prove this by demonstrating that it offers positive outcomes such as those shown in Table 12.1.

Telehealth programs providers usually don't understand how important it is to evaluate their service or why an evaluation should focus on patient outcomes. Outcomes research costs money, and not all telehealth programs can conduct detailed academic research studies. However, it is important for all telehealth programs to be based on sound models for delivering care, models derived from critical evaluation of the clinical components of the care provided. If not, a telehealth program may be unsustainable in today's health care markets, particularly if they demonstrate the same wide variations in practice and variable outcomes that beset so much of the rest of the health care delivery system. As with all new innovations in health care, telehealth is now being put under a harsh financial spotlight by health care purchasers. They are eager to embrace it but only if it delivers the positive outcomes they want to see.

Once an operational telehealth program is established on the basis of a critically evaluated clinical model, this is not the end of outcomes research. The interface of health care information technology systems containing patient data with telehealth systems make low-cost outcomes research possible through analysis of routine data. The results of studies like these can offer outcomes data for the telehealth program to use in negotiating contracts with health care purchasers. They also have a place in quality management initiatives for the program. When health care organizations undertake outcomes research for these reasons, they often rush into it, believing that it is easy, and they confuse process measurement with outcome measurement. Outcomes research involves measuring the health status of patients before and after a health care intervention; that is why it can seem easy. By simply measuring the health status of patients and subtracting the health status before from after the intervention, the outcome can be quantified as shown in Figures 12.2 and 12.3.

Organizations starting to do outcomes research often fail to understand that any outcomes they measure must be clearly attributable to the care they have given. For example, in measuring the survival rates of patients with chest pain in a remote emergency department, better survival rates could suggest that patients with heart attacks are more likely to survive with telehealth support from a cardiologist because therapy is started earlier. To prove that this positive outcome is directly related to the telehealth intervention it is necessary to look in detail at the process of care. Only patients

Table 12.1   Positive Outcomes Telehealth Must Provide

- Reduced costs of care
- Improved access of patients to care
- Increased quality of care at the same or lower cost than alternatives
- Reduced mortality of patients compared to alternatives
- Improved quality of life for patients
- Reduced clinical risk

with mild chest pain may have had a teleconsultation because those with severe and undoubted heart attacks were treated in a resuscitation room where telehealth equipment was not available. Sources of bias such as this can make it seem as though telehealth improves the outcome for patients when it may not. An absolute prerequisite for measuring the outcomes of health care interventions is therefore being able to detail the underlying clinical processes. Clinical standard setting and clinical audit are routine ways of tracking clinical processes.

CLINICAL STANDARD SETTING AND CLINICAL AUDIT

The use of clinical standard setting and clinical audit remains contentious in health care. Clinical standard setting involves agreeing to clear standards detailing how clinical care is delivered. Clinical audit is a systematic process for setting these standards, measuring them, assessing the results, and then feeding back these results to change clinical practice. Some clinicians see these processes as infringements on their individual clinical freedom. Reducing the variations in clinical practice[53] and the resultant inconsistency of outcomes for patients is what provided the rationale for clinical standard setting and clinical audit in the routine delivery of health care services. Telehealth brings us in contact with people who work in industries outside health care who are often amazed that clinical standard setting has been difficult to introduce into health care. A volume manufacturer of computer chips could not remain in business if it tolerated such widespread variations in the quality of the product it produces as is often accepted in health care. Success in the computer industry is based on consistency and attention to detail. This usually requires describing all processes and working practices explicitly. Elsewhere in this book we have given reasons why we believe telehealth should be based on clinical protocols/guidelines. Although patients and diseases may vary, standards of clinical practice should be

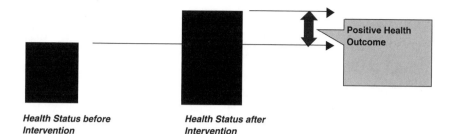

Figure 12.2 A positive outcome from a health care intervention.

consistent. Clinical standard setting and clinical audit are ways to provide this consistency.

Clinical standard setting and clinical audit have been widely introduced into the National Health Service (NHS) in the United Kingdom, and they are now being introduced into health care purchasing.[195] Clinical audit has not gained the same degree of acceptance in the United States. Figure 12.4 shows how clinical standard setting fits into clinical audit as a cycle of quality improvement and health service development. The clinical audit cycle is an ongoing process and allows an organization to look at the quality of service it provides. Analyses can be between different sectors of the same organization over time. It can also be a way of benchmarking with other similar organizations. A practical illustration of how the clinical audit cycle works is devising an audit of the accuracy of clinical diagnosis in a telehealth program.

Step 1. Is There Reason to Identify This As an Area for Audit?

There is evidence in the literature to indicate that the quality of diagnosis in telehealth differs from diagnoses made in face-to-face consultations.[196] Health care purchasers are concerned because some clinicians suggest that a diagnosis made by telehealth is not as accurate as a face-to-face diagnosis. All telehealth programs' clinical risk management policies should always include collecting information about the organization's diagnostic accuracy rate for remote consultation.

It is important to audit regularly the diagnostic accuracy of teleconsultation. This is a quality standard that health care purchasers could reasonably consider imposing on any telehealth program as part of its contract for services.

Step 2. What Clinical Standards Should Be Set, and How Should They Be Set?

The standards needed for a clinical audit depend on the individual requirements of an organization and the questions the audit is intending to answer.

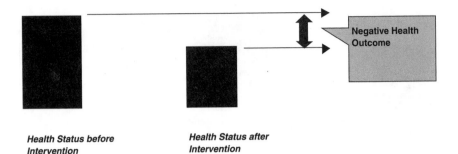

Health Status before
Intervention

Health Status after
Intervention

Figure 12.3   A negative outcome from a health care intervention.

For an audit of diagnostic accuracy in telehealth the standard might reasonably be set as the same accuracy as a face-to-face consultation in making the same diagnosis. The standards should be agreed on by a "standards-setting group." A telehealth program can develop its own standards-setting group or interface with other groups if they exist in health care organizations they work alongside or contract with.

Step 3. Measuring Current Practice Against the Standards That Are Set

Measuring set standards against current clinical practice in an organization should have the rigorous methodology of a research project. The study design of clinical audits will depend on the competency of those designing the audit, the resources available, and the agreement of clinicians and managers to take part in the process. All audits should be assessed internally in the organization against criteria to decide whether or not ethical approval is needed.

We broadly characterize the methodology for clinical audits of diagnostic accuracy in telehealth into two types: *simulation patient audits* and *actual patient audits*. The detailed methodology of these audits can vary. We will outline the differences in methodology in a later section on evidence-based choice. In simulation patient audits, clinicians are tested against prerecorded clinical situations of known diagnoses to assess their accuracy of diagnosis and compare it to a known standard. This is training analogous to an airline pilot in a flight simulator.

In an actual patient audit the diagnostic accuracy of clinicians in telehealth consultations is compared to a random sample or cohort of patients who have a face-to-face consultation as a diagnostic comparator. Typical examples of each type of clinical audit in telehealth are shown below.

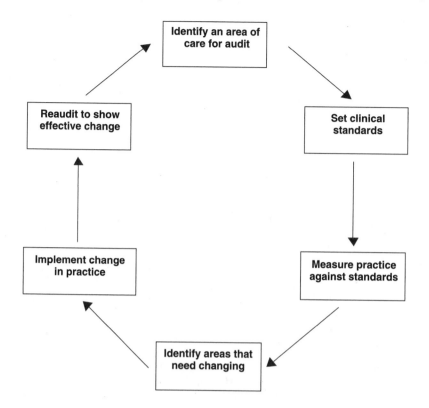

Figure 12.4 The clinical audit cycle.

Examples of Simulated Patient Audits

- ◆ Teledermatology: Still photographs or prerecorded video of patients with already verified dermatological diseases are displayed on a tele-health system for clinicians to make a diagnosis.
- ◆ Teleradiology: x-rays with clearly established diagnoses are displayed for radiologists at the reading site to make diagnoses.
- ◆ Teleneurology: Previously recorded real-time video recordings of patients (e.g., with movement disorders due to known diagnoses) are displayed for the consulting clinicians on the telehealth system for them to make diagnoses.
- ◆ Telepsychiatry: Previously recorded real-time video recordings of patients with known diagnoses of psychiatric disease are conveyed to psychiatrists at the consulting site for them to make diagnoses.
- ◆ Teleneurosurgery: Previous CT scans, x-rays, and/or full-motion videos

of patients with head injuries or other neurosurgical conditions are displayed for clinicians to make an assessment of diagnosis and treatment.

If any patient recordings are used in simulated patient audits, consent from the patient for the recording and their later use for audit must be obtained at the time the original recording is made.

Examples of Actual Patient Audits

- Teledermatology/telepsychiatry/teleotolaryngology: Comparing diagnoses of patients randomly assigned to a telehealth consultation at the consulting center with a face-to-face consultation done at the same center at a later time
- Teledermatology/telepsychiatry/teleotolaryngology: A retrospective audit comparing the eventual diagnosis made on patients after investigation, referral, or treatment, with the initial diagnoses made using telehealth
- Teledermatology/telepsychiatry/teleotolaryngology: Using another experienced clinician to watch the teleconsultation and verify the accuracy of diagnosis

For clinical audit of telehealth, as with any other area of health care, it is essential that clinicians providing the service feel it is clinically relevant to them. Clinicians accept the standard setting process more readily if it is structured using the outline in Table 12.2.

Have a Clear Understanding of Why Clinical Standards Are Being Set and Then Clearly Communicate This to Clinicians

Are clinical guidelines being set for the purposes of clinical outcomes, clinical audit, clinical risk management, or quality improvement or to satisfy the contract requirements of health care purchasers? The reasons for using clinical standards must be quite clear to the clinicians.

Have a Clear Definition of the Standards and How These Are Derived

From where are the clinical standards derived—from international guidelines, (e.g., the World Health Organization [WHO]), government guidelines, professional associations' recommendations, research literature, health care purchaser requirements, or from clinicians themselves?

Institute an Explicit Process for Getting Clinicians' Agreement to Standards

Mechanisms must exist to ensure that the standards have local ownership by clinicians in any organization in which they are to be used, regardless of where they are derived from.

Table 12.2   Suggestions for How to Make Clinical Standard Setting and Clinical Audit Work in Practice Using Telehealth

- Have a clear understanding of why clinical standards are being set and clearly communicate this to clinicians.
- Have a clear definition of the standards and how these are derived.
- Institute an explicit process for getting the agreement of clinicians to standards.
- Make the clinical audit an efficient process for measuring standards, with a robust methodology that can deliver meaningful results.
- Make the process of giving results of audits back to clinicians simple, and do this to get their feedback before releasing any results of the audit.
- Have a clear process to use information gained to improve practice.
- Make sure that the need to reaudit once the change in practice has been instituted was made clear at the beginning of the clinical audit process.

Devise an Efficient Process for Measuring Standards, With a Robust Methodology That Can Deliver Meaningful Results

Clinicians are busy, and their time with patients is precious. Wherever possible, data for clinical audit should be collected as part of the routine data-collecting process. The fact that telehealth systems are usually difficult to interface with clinical information systems can make replication of data collection necessary. This is frustrating for patients and clinicians and should be avoided whenever possible. It is important to feed back interim results to clinicians as audits are progressing. All too often clinicians can feel that data collection in health care is "feeding the beast," and they do not get data feedback to help them in practice. Clinicians are scientifically trained. They will have no respect for the clinical audit process if they suspect the methodology of an audit is so flawed that the results will be meaningless. An area where difficulties and confusion with clinical audit can arise is in qualitative studies. Clinicians who are typically trained in quantitative analyses can find these difficult because there are no hard data.

Make the Process of Feeding Results Back to Clinicians Simple, and Do This to Get Their Feedback Before Releasing Any Results of the Audit

Clinical audit can feel threatening to clinicians. The traditional culture in health care has been one of working in isolation as autonomous professionals without a process to compare one individual's results (outcomes) with another's. If audits are seen as pitting individuals against each other in competition or as a witch hunt for bad clinicians, then it is threatening. Clinical audits should be concerned with organizational learning and improving overall clinical performance. Clinical audit results should therefore be fed back to clinicians with this in mind. If the clinical service does not meet the standards set, what does this mean? It could be that the set standards are not relevant. It could be that the service is substandard. These possibilities should be discussed with clinicians first and any changes to practice agreed to in advance.

Have a Clear Process for Using the Information Gained to Improve Practice

When clinical audits suggest that clinical practice needs to change, almost invariably the recommendations are about how teams rather than individuals alter the way they work. Therefore, they usually require training and professional development to implement any changes. The change management process involved in implementing changes after a clinical audit requires sensitivity to the clinical situation and the team of individuals concerned. The result required is an optimally performing clinical team, not a dysfunctional situation where patient care is adversely affected. In this respect clinical audit and clinical risk management are very closely linked, as we will describe later in this chapter.

Make Sure That the Need to Reaudit Once the Change in Practice Has Been Instituted Was Made Clear at the Beginning of the Clinical Audit Process

When a clinical service meets the clinical audit standards set for it, there is no need to change clinical practice. The audit will not have to be repeated unless it forms a part of a regularly repeated cycle of clinical audits. If a clinical service fails to meet the set standards, then it must be repeated once the corrective changes in clinical practice have been made. It must be repeated to ensure that care of patients has been improved and for clinical risk management reasons. If a health care organization audits a service and finds a fault, then fails to rectify this fault and harm comes to a patient as a result, the organization is likely to find itself legally culpable. Clinicians must understand at the start of an audit that the process may involve clinical change and reaudit.

CLINICAL RISK MANAGEMENT

Clinical standard setting and clinical audit in health care overlap with clinical risk management. Clinical risk management had its origin in the United States in the 1970s and 1980s, prompted by increasing litigation from errors in clinical judgment. It has been widely introduced into health trusts in the United Kingdom since 1996 as part of the arrangements for the Clinical Negligence Scheme for Trusts. Covering the costs of litigation adds significantly to cost inflation in health care. With improvements in computing, sophisticated claims databases have been developed. These databases show areas in health care service delivery where consistently high risks of litigation exist, as in obstetric and emergency care. Yet only a small proportion of the large number of clinical errors in health care eventually result in litigation.[197] In the United States as many as 180,000 deaths and 1.3 million injuries each year may be related to receiving health care.[198] In Australia, 16% of hospital admissions include an adverse event, and there are 14,000 preventable deaths per year.[199] Clinical risk management is a proactive approach to the very real problem of clinical errors in health care, and it involves elements shown in Table 12.3.

Monitoring Complaints in Telehealth Programs

Telehealth organizations must focus on the care they give to patients. It therefore makes sense that they respond to any complaints made by patients and relatives about the quality of services they receive. Apart from the direct concern about giving patients the best-quality care there are three reasons associated with clinical risk management that a telehealth program should deal efficiently with complaints:

- Identifying areas where potential clinical errors can occur
- Reducing the risk of litigation
- Meeting any organizational standards for complaints

Telehealth programs often provide services at the interface of several different parts of the health care system, such as primary care and acute hospital care. It is imperative for telehealth programs to actively seek feedback from patients on the service provided. This feedback must involve establishing a clear *complaints procedure* for the organization, with a regular reporting system to the senior executive team. The reporting system should include a database of clinical complaints. The function of this complaints database is to record details of who made a complaint, when the event happened, and where the care this relates to was given. Regular analysis of these data can identify if complaints are clustering in certain parts of the service. When the senior management team takes complaints seriously, it sets an example for the rest of the organization. The complaints procedure then serves as a direct stimulus to improve patient care. High numbers of complaints clustering in a particular part of the organization may be the first indication of poor-quality clinical care. Investigation and corrective action can be taken and may prevent avoidable adverse incidents involving patients later.

Table 12.3   Strategies for Clinical Risk Management

- Monitor patient complaints as an indication of areas of risk.
- Deal fully and sympathetically with patients complaints.
- Establish an incident reporting system and monitor all adverse incidents.
- Establish clinical standards in areas of known high clinical risk and monitor these on a regular basis.
- Establish a database of clinical incidents and clinical claims.
- Establish a claims management system.
- Train clinical staff and managers in awareness of clinical risk.

Deal Fully and Sympathetically With Patients' Complaints

Only a minority of patients who have suffered an adverse clinical incident while receiving care take this further and proceed to litigation against a health care organization. When the cases of patients or relatives litigating against health care organizations are reviewed, the reason a patient embarks on the path of litigation is frequently that his/her complaint was not adequately dealt with at an early stage. Telehealth programs must not be complacent about the possibility of litigation just because there is no significant litigation record currently associated with telehealth. The current levels of telehealth transactions are low. Much of telehealth is taking place under the protective umbrella of grant-funded projects. Litigation cases typically take up to 7 years to work through the system. The recent upsurge in telehealth in the United States and the United Kingdom is less than 7 years old. It is therefore not surprising that telehealth has yet to build up a litigation history. It makes sense for telehealth programs to learn the lesson of other areas of health care and manage clinical complaints from patients fully and sympathetically.

Establish an Incident Reporting System and Monitor All Adverse Incidents

A critical incident reporting system is an important part of a clinical risk management policy that telehealth programs should adopt. Adverse incidents include

- Harm to patients
- Infectious disease monitoring
- Harm to staff
- Equipment failure or damage

Prescribing in telehealth is an area of high potential risk.[200] In a general health care setting, a rate of drug prescription error of 3 per 1,000 is quoted, and half of these errors could harm patients.[201] In telehealth, where consultations are taking place between specialist and nonspecialist centers, there often are no clear procedures to detail how prescribing is done other than as telephone conversations. Telehealth consultations can involve advice about prescribing unfamiliar medications at remote sites. Health care organizations have their own "adverse event" reporting systems that should include prescribing errors. It is a simple managerial task to link these adverse event reporting systems to a telehealth program. A telehealth organization should have its own adverse event reporting system linked to the senior management team. This system should include policies and procedures for deciding how to deal with a member of the clinical staff who is involved in an adverse clinical event.

The current advice in clinical risk management circles is for organizations to adopt "no fault" adverse event reporting systems wherever possible. No fault means that unless an adverse event is particularly serious, then staff should not be punished for reporting when one has occurred. A no-fault system is thought to make it easier to establish where problems exist with clinical quality. A punitive system of reporting may discourage staff from reporting problems at an early stage and possibly preventing a major incident occurring later. Earlier knowledge of adverse events can indicate areas of poor clinical quality in which the risk of a major incident is high.

Establish Clinical Standards in Areas of Known High Clinical Risk and Monitor These on a Regular Basis

Instead of waiting for an adverse event or major incident, clinical standard setting, clinical audit, and clinical risk management are ways of preempting this. In the initial stages of a telehealth program the initiators of the program are often clear about roles, responsibilities, and clinical protocols. As the program expands, staff turnover and the employment of temporary staff may mean that the initial clear understanding of roles, responsibilities, and protocols gets lost in the organization. Clear clinical procedures and protocols/guidelines are ways to help guard against this. Standard setting and clinical audit are processes to help ensure the training of new staff and reduce clinical risk. The areas in which standards should be set and audited will vary from organization to organization depending on where clinical risk is thought most probable to exist. An important area for all organizations to concentrate on is the recording of clinical information in the case records. Without an integrated clinical record the patient's clinical notes are a major area of risk for telehealth organizations. Setting standards for record keeping and then monitoring them is a particularly important area for all telehealth programs.

Establish a Database of Clinical Incidents and Clinical Claims

With the myriad of tasks associated with establishing a telehealth program, a database for clinical complaints, clinical incidents, and clinical claims can seem irrelevant. Large health care organizations such as academic teaching centers and general hospitals are finding it difficult to introduce management tools such as clinical audit and clinical risk management because they are used to accepting the range of clinical practice variation that exists. These variations in practice are reinforced by historical precedent in these organizations and perpetuated by the attitude of clinicians who are used to being autonomous. As telehealth is being introduced, there are opportunities to incorporate clinical guidelines and methods of audit and risk management into routine clinical practice. The processes of clinical audit and clinical risk management are relatively worthless as managerial tools if the data from them are not recorded on relational or object-linked databases.

Establish a Claims Management System

An important adjunct to a clinical risk management program is a claims management system. In general health care, as opposed to telehealth programs, managing claims for litigation is a significant managerial task for an organization. Efficient claims management should begin with the management of clinical complaints. For stand-alone telehealth programs it is worthwhile to consider establishing a claims management process before they receive their first claim against the service.

Train Clinical Staff and Managers in Awareness of Clinical Risk

The most important aspect of clinical risk management in health care is the training of clinicians and managers. It is impossible to think of creating processes to set standards for all clinical care and monitoring them. The end result would probably be clinicians who spend all their time measuring and monitoring and have no time to look after patients. The importance of clinical risk management is in establishing a culture in which clinicians and managers are vigilant for areas of potential clinical risk. Clinicians are usually aware of clinical risk at an individual level. Rarely have they been trained to think of clinical risk in organizational terms. The object of clinical risk management is to create a corporate ethos in which people think about clinical risk and improving care to patients. We have indicated how a clinical risk management program can help reduce litigation. However, its primary purpose is to improve patient care. Telehealth is opening up new ideas about how to deliver health care and consequently new dangers. The way to provide high-quality care to patients and reduce the risk of litigation to a telehealth program is to recognize these dangers proactively and guard against them, not to wait until patients are injured and the organization faces possible legal redress.

The training of staff in clinical risk management in a telehealth program has two important principles. The first principle is that all staff working in the organization be made aware of the general principles of clinical risk management. This includes what it can achieve and how it can do this. The second important principle is that staff are trained in the actual policies and procedures that apply within the telehealth organization and other organizations with which they must interface. It is important for the management of clinical risk to designate roles and responsibilities clearly.

EVIDENCE-BASED HEALTH CARE
AND EVIDENCE-BASED CHOICE

Evidence-based health care is an approach to decision making in which the clinician uses the best evidence available on the effectiveness of treatments to plan the management of patients.[202] Outcomes research, clinical audit, and clinical risk management all fit into the bigger picture of evidence-based health care. Evidence-based health care currently poses two big challenges for telehealth. The first challenge is to provide definitive evidence that delivering health care remotely is clinically effective and cost-effective. The second is to find evidence that the health care interventions on which telehealth services are based are themselves effective.

The theory of evidence-based health care is clear and a welcome change aimed at ensuring quality and consistency in health care practice. The practicalities of how evidence-based health care can be implemented within health care systems are less clear. "Evidence" must be a currency to work in the health care system. The evidence must have a recognized worth, a stable value, and free convertibility among areas of care. Decimalization of the currency in the United Kingdom in the early 1970s and the forthcoming single European currency show how introducing a new monetary currency means agreeing to new standards on a vast scale. Even with money, where these standards are agreed on, it is a major logistical exercise to introduce a new currency. In health care it is not clear how the immense logistical exercise of gathering evidence of effectiveness and implementing it into practice will be accomplished.

A big problem is that there is no widely accepted new currency that clinicians will freely accept as evidence of effectiveness. The old currencies some clinicians used resemble a system of barter rather than coinage, anecdote and habit playing a major role in determining clinical care over consistent evaluation. Telehealth is a new area of health care, and it is starting with a relatively clean slate in terms of the models of practice it uses. We strongly urge telehealth programs to devise protocols for care and set standards for practice based on scientific evidence. Then they should monitor the practice of telehealth and use these data to contribute to the body of knowledge about the effectiveness of telehealth. Standards for how telehealth is practiced must be set now, at the outset, rather than being introduced later. If telehealth joins the general hodgepodge of health care, where only 20% of interventions are known to be effective, it will face great problems in acceptance.

The current gold standard in evidence-based medicine is the double-blind, randomized, controlled trial (RCT). RCTs are expensive, and can take large numbers of patients/controls and many years to produce definitive results. Most health care interventions have not been subjected to RCTs to show their effectiveness, and the logistics of how, if ever, this will be done for all interventions in the future is hazy. In the meantime, clinicians, patients, and managers use a variety of sources of evidence to gauge the effectiveness and appropriateness of a health care intervention. The US Preventive Services Task Force[68] adapted work done by the Canadian Task Force on the Periodic Health Examination[203–206] and devised a systematic way of looking at the evidence of health care interventions and rating their quality. Their 5-point scale is shown in Table 12.4.

A major growth area for telehealth is the use of the Internet by patients to assess information about health and health care interventions. We have mentioned the potential problems associated with the patient having many pages of Internet material to query their doctor about during a consultation. There is no easy way for physician and patient to use Internet-derived

Table 12.4   A Scale to Assessing the Quality of Evidence[68]

Rating	Rationale for rating
I	Evidence obtained from at least one properly designed randomized controlled trial
II-1	Evidence obtained from well-designed controlled trials without randomization
II-2	Evidence obtained from well-designed cohort or case-control analytic studies, preferably from more than one center or research group
II-3	Evidence obtained from multiple time series with or without the intervention; dramatic results in uncontrolled experiments
III	Opinions of respected authorities, based on clinical evidence, descriptive studies, or reports of expert committees

health information as a currency in negotiating joint decisions about what course of action (or inaction) is most suitable for a patient to take. It seems unlikely in the short term that all patients will reach the stage of being able to critically access the quality of scientific evidence from a research journal for themselves, although many can. What is required is a commonly accepted way for patients and clinicians (in both allopathic and nonallopathic branches of medicine) to view the evidence of an intervention's effectiveness and use this as a currency to help exchange ideas about the correct clinical decision in any circumstance. One way this could be done is shown in Table 12.5, a scale we have adapted from one described by the US Preventive Services Task Force[68] to assess preventive interventions.

An agreed-to grading system and means of applying this to information recommending options for investigation, management, and treatment in health care would offer a way for patients and clinicians to use information objectively to help make the right choices, choices that work for the individual subjective situation of patients needing to make a decision about their health. The growth in Internet-based health services involving information and treatment will present a future in health care that is about evidence-based choice and will refocus the delivery of health care services back on the patient, where it properly belongs.

Making telehealth a reality requires the reengineering of health care delivery systems. These systems involve attitudinal changes in health care professionals and patients as well as the implementation and integration of a

Table 12.5   Strength of Recommendation for an Intervention

Grade of recommendation	Rationale for the grade
A	There is good evidence to recommend the investigation, treatment, or course of action proposed in the evidence being presented.
B	There is fair evidence to recommend the investigation, treatment, or course of action proposed in the evidence being presented.
C	There is poor evidence to recommend the investigation, treatment, or course of action proposed in the evidence being presented.
D	There is fair evidence to advise against recommending the investigation, treatment, or course of action proposed in the evidence being presented.
E	There is good evidence to advise against recommending the investigation, treatment, or course of action proposed in the evidence being presented.

complex information-and-communications network. Many people express frustration at what they see as the slow pace of telehealth development over the past 8 years. They know what it can do and vent at why it is not doing it now. As we have mentioned on several occasions in this book, the challenge for telehealth is in developing revenue streams and making real inroads into the private health care sector.

In concluding this book and considering a vision for the next 5 years, it is useful to look back at the development of the Internet. The Internet was originally conceived in the late 1960s as a means of connecting large computers serving U.S. Department of Defense installations. The next stage was bringing in academic centers and the true embryonic Internet as we know it began to grow. This partnership between academia and the military sponsored and fostered by congress and successive administrations resulted in a number of discrete products that underpin the Internet now. These products include:

- Packet switching of data
- File transfer
- Remote log-in
- E-mail
- Domain naming

It seems unlikely in retrospect that private investment could have developed the Internet at the same pace. The Internet (Internet 1) was passed to the private sector in 1995. This represented a 30-year evolutionary partnership between the military, academia, and then the private sector. The next-generation Internet is now under development using a similar public/private model. It is often difficult for the private sector to invest in projects that have a long cycle in terms of return on investment. Recent trends in the stock market mean that Wall Street now looks for a 1–2 year timeline for its return on investments. Yet, few would now suggest that the Internet should not have been developed.

In many ways the development of the Internet has many parallels to the current situation in telemedicine. Government investment in the military, rural health care, schools and libraries, and the Veterans Health Administration in the form of grants to large academic centers is building the infrastructure and model that will migrate across into the private sector. This investment is also encouraging hardware and software developers to create the tools of information technology and the communications infrastructure which will support telehealth. Our message to people who feel impatient with the pace of development is to remind them of the scale of what needs to be achieved.

Many telehealth projects are still at the level of being point to point. The quantum leap now necessary for telehealth requires a jump to telehealth networks. It is these networks that will make it possible to

- Get immediate access to specialist care
- Move surplus health care capacity around the network
- Reduce costs
- Improve access
- Educate health care consumers
- Offer real choices to patients

We believe, as do so many others, that these changes are going to happen. The great challenge is in the clinical and organization changes that are the foundations on which the networks must be grown.

End Note

Telehealth is an exciting area to watch for new developments. It is the current focus of a social revolution at least as great as that created by the Internet and e-commerce on trade and industry. Events in this world are moving so quickly that the players, the ideas, and the technology are all rapidly evolving. Constants are the underlying currents driving these changes and the tides and barriers affecting where events are likely to be taken by them. Throughout this book we have often alluded to these currents, tides, and barriers. We felt this End Note necessary because when reviewing the book for the final time before publication we realized how so many of the events we speculated on months previously had already happened.

The most striking change has been the phenomenon that is the ongoing growth of health information on-line. We are amazed by the rapid emergence of major health care information portals and such a myriad of new and different Web sites. The business model for many of these "health information resources" is based on attracting sponsorship or advertising revenue from organizations interested in direct sales to health care consumers. Often these are large established organizations in health care retailing such as the pharmaceutical industry and herb wholesalers. This movement is creating some interesting paradoxes. The large pharmaceutical companies are moving from advertising and sales that target physicians toward a strategy of direct marketing to consumers. The Internet is the ideal vehicle to use to reach out directly to the consumer. However, as the size of the Web community has exploded, it is increasingly difficult to reach the consumer, who now has an Aladdin's cave of choice of health-information sites on the Web. Many of the Internet health care portals have content that is an inch deep and a mile wide, making the jewels in the cave costume, not gem stones.

Consequently, many health care Web sites are desperate for content and exposure. Internet companies are now spending vast amounts of money to market their Web sites using conventional advertising channels. The paradox for companies who are targeted as sponsors and advertisers of Internet Web sites is that their presence on the site can in itself provide content and legitimacy. Who therefore should be paying whom? Should the Web sites be paying the pharmaceutical companies to come onto their sites? The situation of Internet health consumer information sites is therefore in a bizarre and transitory state. It is a battle in cyberspace almost worthy of a *Star Wars* story. As the various forces vie to create their empires it is less clear what their agendas mean in relation to ordinary individuals and their health. Currently the individual Web traveler seems targeted as a passive consumer. S/he is viewed as a bird of passage on the Internet to entrap and then to peddle her/him a variety of pills, potions, and on-line consultation. This hard sell in cyberspace is largely unregulated and usually does not give the consumer access to an unbiased evidence base from which to make informed decisions. It is easy to draw the analogies with a century ago when medicine men in the Wild West hawked their questionable wares of brightly colored liquids in bottles with garish names. The covered wagons of what many now see as contemporary snake-oil salesmen in cyberspace are drawn by applets instead of mules. Because health information sites and pharmaceutical supply has been unable to self-regulate we foresee a major attempt by government to do so. This is a pity because great sites with integrity and concern about patients are currently suffering from the activities of those who are less scrupulous.

Although most major health care providers have a substantial Web presence, there has been little movement toward directly providing health care to consumers via the Web. A move away from low-volume/high-cost applications toward high-volume/low-cost applications such as home care is now well established. The barrier of licensure clearly remains a clear obstacle to the direct delivery of clinical services to patients using telehealth. Where health care providers are making tremendous use of the Internet is in relation to medical records and the distribution of medical images. With secure encryption and the developing sophistication of Web technology, it is now possible to link institutions and share records in an unprecedented way. The major influences on health care providers will therefore be:

+ Attempts to change licensure laws
+ Privacy and confidentiality regulation relating to telehealth and electronic records
+ The rapidly diminishing cost of the technology

It was only a short time ago that the favored solution to most societal problems seemed to be government regulation. The traditional answers to many of the questions we have raised throughout this book would have been to lobby for legislation. It is less clear how legislation can keep up with the pace of change. Many legislators are unaware of the issues because they are not savvy about the technology. Before we consider legislation and telehealth further we predict a rapid change in the use of the Internet by politicians and legislators. A cardinal rule of politics is that you have to be where the people are. Not only the people but their cars, refrigerators, and toasters will be on the Web. A problem for legislators is that development of the Web is like a chemical reaction. Change the amount of heat or the chemical constituents and the reaction could stop or reverse. Now back to how legislation can influence the Web. The situation is complex in the literal sense and also because complexity theory, not linear dynamics, applies as the Web involves global issues and huge societal change. One option may be that legal rights on parts of the Web may resemble an aspect of law in ancient Rome. In Rome there were parts of the city where the roads were not straight and narrow. These areas where the roads curved and there were bumps were called the "red-light districts." In these places "off the straight and narrow" Roman law did not apply. It may be that there will be no secure legal answers to everything that is possible in relation to health (or anything else) on the Web. As citizens of a particular country we may have information that Web sites are obliged to inform us about where our laws apply and we have legal redress. If we choose to go outside this zone of safety we will be off the "straight and narrow" and there will be no sure means to pursue legal redress. In fact this is the case already. A person in Colorado buying Viagra from New Zealand has no surety of the product in terms of what it contains and at what dose. This person is purchasing a prescription-only drug and may have no easy means of redress if he has a heart attack on Viagra. Is the Colorado consumer purchasing illegally or the New Zealand supplier selling illegally? What about the Internet Services Provider? Is it aiding and abetting a potentially illegal transaction? In the health care provision vacuum we are describing the void may be filled by coalitions of lawyers from different countries creating an interoperability of legal systems through partnerships. We will have to wait and see.

We want to finish this book back where we began and where we feel its focus should be—on the patient. What of the patient? We are optimistic about the future and how the knowledge revolution will change health care. We believe that ultimately the coupling of knowledge engineering to health care delivery will increase access, reduce costs, and improve quality. Our premise for making this statement stems from looking back at the parallel concerns at the time of the industrial revolution and subsequent events. How will positive change come about? We cannot say precisely because there are many routes it could take. Our health care system and the Internet interact in a complex adaptive system and as a result produce the changes we see and those we anticipate. There are underlying drivers and no overarching master plan. Despite having no clear map we believe the way forward is surprisingly simple and is no different from that in Hippocrates's time: *Remember the patient, and first and foremost do no harm.* By following these simple rules we believe in the future of the health care system, the growth of telehealth, the involvement of physicians and other health care professionals, and the disappearance of any cyber snake-oil sellers along the way.

References

1. Bashshur R, Sanders J, Shannon G. *Telemedicine Theory and Practice.* Springfield, IL: Charles C Thomas; 1997.
2. Wootton R. Telemedicine fad or future? *Lancet.* 1995;345:73–74.
3. Reid J. *A Telemedicine Primer: Understanding the issues.* Billings, Mt.: Innovative Medical Communications; 1996.
4. Antezana F. Telehealth and telemedicine will henceforth be part of the strategy for health for all. Internet, 1997; http://www.who.ch//
5. *Webster's Seventh New Collegiate Dictionary.* Springfield, Mass.: G. & C., Merriam; 1971.
6. McKeown T. *The role of medicine.* Oxford: Blackwell; 1979.
7. Aronson SH. The Lancet on the telephone 1876–1975. *Med Hist.* 1977; 21:60–87.
8. Anonymous letter to the editor. *Lancet.* 1897; 819.
9. Wittson CL, Benschotter R. Two-way television: Helping the medical center reach out. *Am J Psychiatry.* 1972;129:136–139.
10. DeBakey M. Telemedicine has now come of age. *Telemedicine Journal.* 1995; 1:3–4.
11. Bashshur R. Critical issues in telemedicine. *Telemedicine Journal.* 1997;3: 113–126.
12. Bird, K. *Teleconsultation: A New Health Information Exchange System: Third Annual Report to the Veterans Administration, Boston, MA.* Boston: Massachusetts General Hospital; 1971.
13. Cawthon MA, Goeringer F, Telepak RJ, et al. Preliminary assessment of computer tomography and satellite teleradiology from Operation Desert Storm. *Invest Radiol.* 1991;26:854–857.
14. Pedersen S, Hartviksen G. Teleconsultation of patients with otorhinolaryngologic conditions. *Arch Otolaryngol Head and Neck.* 1994;120:133–136.
15. Nordrum I, Engum B, Rinde E, et al. Remote frozen section service: A telepathology project in northern Norway. *Hum Pathol.* 1991;22:514–518.

16. Viitanen J, Sund T, Rinde E, et al. Nordic teleradiology development. *Comput Methods Programs Biomed.* 1992;37:273–277.
17. Pedersen S, Hartviksen G. Telemedisin—en oversikt [Telemedicine—a review]. *Tidsskr Nor Laegeforen.* 1994;114:1212–1214.
18. Brecht RM, Gray CL, Peterson C, Youngblood B. The University of Texas Medical Branch, Texas Department of Criminal Justice Telemedicine Project: Findings from the first year of operation. *Telemedicine Journal.* 1996;2:25–35.
19. Anno BJ. Health care for prisoners. *JAMA.* 1993;269:633–634.
20. Adams JB, Grigsby RK. The Georgia state telemedicine program: Initiation, design and plans. *Telemedicine Journal.* 1995;1:227–236.
21. Hassol A, Gaumer G, Grigsby J, Mintzer C, Puskin D, Brunswick M. Rural telemedicine: A national snapshot. *Telemedicine Journal.* 1996;2:43–48.
22. Hassol A, Irvin C, Gaumer G, Puskin D, Mintzer C, Grigsby J. Rural applications of telemedicine. *Telemedicine Journal.* 1997;3:215–225.
23. Allen A. Editorial. *Telemedicine Today.* 1997;5(5):5.
24. Grigsby B, Allen A. Fourth annual telemedicine program review. *Telemedicine Today.* 1997;August 1997, pp. 30–38.
25. Heagarty MC. From house calls to telephone calls. *Am J Public Health.* 1978;68:14–15.
26. Hallam L. You've got a lot to answer for, Mr Bell: A review of the use of the telephone in primary care. *Family Practice.* 1989;6:47–57.
27. Nouilhan P, Dutau G. Le pediatre et le telephone [The pediatrician and the telephone]. *Arch Pediatr.* 1995;2:891–894.
28. Pert JC, Furth TW, Katz HP. A 10-year experience in pediatric after-hours telecommunications. *Curr Opin Pediatr.* 1996;8:181–187.
29. Sola JE, Scherer LR, Haller-JA J, Colombani PM, Papa PA, Paidas CN. Criteria for safe cost-effective pediatric trauma triage: Prehospital evaluation and distribution of injured children. *J Pediatr Surg.* 1994;29:738–741.
30. Sturtz GS, Brown RB. Concerning A.G. Bell's invention. *Clin Pediatr.* 1969; 8:378–380.
31. Curtis P, Talbot A. The telephone in primary care. *Community Health.* 1981; 6:194–203.
32. Mendenhall RC, Butler JC. *Medical Practice in the United States: Special Report.* Robert Wood Johnson Foundation; Princton N.J.: 1981.
33. Office of Population Censuses and Surveys. *General Household Survey.* London: HMSO; 1985.
34. Evens S, Curtis P, Talbot ABC, Smart A. Characteristics and perceptions of after hours callers. *Family Practice.* 1985;2:10–16.
35. Greenlick MR, Freeborn DK, Gambill GL. Determinants of medical care utilization: The use of the telephone for reporting symptoms. *Med Care.* 1973;11:121–134.
36. Weiss JE, Greenlick MR. Determinants of medical care utilization: The effect of social class and distance on contacts with the medical care system. *Med Care.* 1970;8:456–462.

37. Freeman TR. A study of telephone prescriptions in family practice. *J Fam Pract.* 1980;10:857–862.
38. Ott JE, Bellaire J, Machotka P, Moon JB. Patient management by telephone by child health associates and pediatric house officers. *J Med Educ.* 1974;49:596–600.
39. Perrin EC, Goodman HC. Telephone management of acute paediatric illnesses. *N Engl J Med.* 1978;298:130–135.
40. Nickerson HJ, Biechler L, Witte F. How dependable is diagnosis and management of earache by telephone? *Clin Paed (Phila).* 1975;14:920–923.
41. Katz HP, Posen J, Mushlin AI. Quality assessment of a telephone care system utilizing non-physician personnel. *Am Heart J.* 1978;68:31–38.
42. Bhopal JS, Bhopal RS. Outcome and duration of telephone consultations in a general practice. *J R Coll Gen Pract.* 1988;38:566.
43. Levy JC, Strasser PH, Lamb GA, Rosenkrans J, Friedman M, Kaplan D. Survey of telephone encounters in three pediatric practice sites. *Public Health Rep.* 1980;95:324–328.
44. Curtis P, Evens S, Berolzheimer N, Beery M. *Telephone Medicine.* Boston: Health Services Consortium Inc.; 1987.
45. Brown JL. *Telephone Medicine.* St Louis: CV Mosby; 1980.
46. Group Health of Puget Sound. *Nurse's Guide to Telephone Health Care.* Baltimore: Williams and Wilkins; 1984.
47. Flannery MT, Moses GA, Cykert S, et al. Telephone management training in internal medicine residencies: A national survey of program directors. *Acad Med.* 1995;70:1138–1141.
48. Hannis MD, Hazard RL, Rothschild M, Elnicki DM, Keyserling TC, DeVellis RF. Physician attitudes regarding telephone medicine. *J Gen Intern Med.* 1996;11:678–683.
49. Eisenthal S, Lazare A. Evaluation of the initial interview in a walk-in clinic: The patient's perspective on a "customer approach." *J Nerv Ment Dis.* 1976; 162:169–176.
50. Evens S, Curtis P, Talbot A, Baer C, Smart A. Characteristics and perceptions of after-hours callers. *Family Practice.* 1985;2:10–16.
51. MedicineNet™ Home Page. Consumer Medhelp. Internet, 1998.
52. Consumer Medhelp. Internet, 1998. http:www.consumermedhelp.com
53. Saunders D, Coulter A, McPherson K. *Variation in the Hospital Admission Rates: A Review of the Literature.* London: King's Fund; 1989.
54. Takizawa M, Sone S, Aoki J, et al. [High-speed/high resolution teleradiology system based on university microwave network]. *Nippon Igaku Hoshasen Gakkai Zasshi.* 1994;54:1285–1293.
55. Telemedicine bibliography. Internet, 1998. http://www.nlm.nih.gov/pubs/cbm/telembib.html
56. Medline. Internet, 1998.
57. Healthfinder. Internet, 1998. http://healthfinder.gov
58. Food and Drug Adminstration. Internet, 1998. http://www.fda.gov/fdahomepage.html

59. Health Care Financing Administration. Internet, 1998. http://www.hcfa.gov/

60. US Department of Health and Human Services. Internet, 1998. http://www.os.dhss.gov/

61. Flory J (ed). *1997 Healthcare Guide to the Internet.* Santa Barbara, Calif.: COR Healthcare Resources; published four times yearly. http://www.mednet-i.com

62. Advantage Health Plan. Internet, 1998. http://inet1.healthcareadvantage.com/index.html

63. American Association of Health Plans. Health Plan Associations. Internet, 1998. http://www.aahp.org/

64. About Group Health Cooperatve. Medical Groups. Internet, 1998. http://www.ghc.org/about_gh/contents.html

65. Columbia Park Healthcare System. Internet, 1998. http://www.photobooks.com/~cphs/

66. HospitalWeb. Internet, 1998. http://neuro-www.mgh.harvard.edu/hospital-web.nclk

67. Barry M, Fowler A, Mulley A. Patient reactions to a program to facilitate patient participation in treatment decisions for benign prostatic hyperplasia. *Medical Care.* 1998;33:771–82.

68. US Preventive Services Task Force. *Guide to Clinical Preventive Services. An Assessment of the Effectiveness of 169 Interventions.* Baltimore: Williams and Wilkins; 1989.

69. Darkins A. Evidence-based medicine dream or reality? In: Spiers J, ed. *Dilemmas in Modern Health Care.* London: Social Market Foundation; 1997:33–46.

70. Eng TR, Gustafson DH, eds. *Wired for Health and Well-Being: The Emergence of Interactive Health Communication.* Washington D.C.: Science Panel on Interactive Communication and Health, USDHHS Office of Public Health and Science. 1999.

71. Holden G, Bearison D, Rode DC, Rosenberg G, Fishman M. Evaluating the effects of a virtual environment (Starbright World) with hospitalized children. *Res Soc Work Practice.* 1999;9:365–382.

72. Jones WHS. *Hippocrates.* London: GP Putnam's Sons, New York (In Greek with English translation); 1923.

73. Peabody FW. The care of the patient. *JAMA.* 1923;88:877.

74. Feinstein AR. *Clinical Judgememt.* Baltimore: Williams and Wilkins; 1967;24–25.

75. Abramovitch H, Schwartz E. Three stages of medical dialogue. *Theor Med.* 1996;17:175–187.

76. Barcia D. Ethical aspects of the doctor-patient relationship. *Eur J Med.* 1993;2:301–304.

77. Dewberry-GP J. Say no to government control of patient care. *Postgrad Med.* 1994;95:27–30.

78. La PJ. Anticipated changes in the doctor-patient relationship in the managed care and managed competition of the Health Security Act of 1993. *Arch Fam Med.* 1994;3:665–671.

79. Perkel RL. Ethics and managed care. *Med Clin North Am.* 1996;80:263–278.

80. Lawrence RS. The physician's perception of health care. *J R Soc Med.* 1994;87 (suppl 22):11–14.
81. The United States Information Infrastructure Task Force. *The National Information Infrastructure.* 1993, Washington D.C.: Author.
82. Darkins A. The Future of Telemedicine in the NHS. The Health Summary. *National Health Service Policymaker.* 1997;12(5).
83. Lazare A, Putman SM, Lipkin M. Three functions of the medical interview. In: Lipkin M, Putman SM, Lazare A, eds. *The Medical Interview.* New York: Springer-Verlag; 1995:3–19.
84. Seidel V, Seidel R. Health care and medical care in the United States. In: Conrad P, Kern R, eds. *Sociology of Health and Illness: Critical Perspectives.* New York: St Martin's Press; 1986:257–271.
85. Vickery DM, Kalmer H, Lowry D, Constatine, M, Wright, M, Loren W. Effect of a self-care education program on medical visits. *JAMA.* 1983;250: 2952–2956.
86. Vickery DM, Lynch WD. Demand management: Enabling patients to use medical care appropriately. *Journal of Occupational and Environmental Medicine.* 1995;37:551–557.
87. Freemon B, Negrete VF, Davis M, Korsch BM. Gaps in doctor-patient communication: Doctor patient interaction analysis. *Pediatr Res.* 1971;5:298–311.
88. Beckman HB, Frankel RM. The effect of physician behavior on the collection of data. *Ann Intern Med.* 1984;101:692–696.
89. Hampton JR, Harrison MJG, Mitchell JRA, Prichard JS, Seymour C. Relative contribtions of history-taking, physical examination, and laboratory examination to diagnosis and management of medical outpatients. *Br Med J.* 1975;2:486–489.
90. Sandler G. The importance of the history in the medical clinic and the cost of unnecessary tests. *Am Heart J.* 1980;100:928–931.
91. Kassirer JP. Teaching medicine by iterative hypothesis testing. *N Engl J Med.* 1983;309:893–900.
92. Nitzkin J, Zhu N, Marier R. Reliability of telemedicine examination. *Telemedicine Journal.* 1997;3:141–157.
93. Darkins A, Dearden CH, Rocke LG, Martin JB, Sibson L, Wootton R. An evaluation of telemedical support for a minor treatment center. *Journal of Telemedicine and Telecare.* 1996;2:93–99.
94. American College of Radiology. *ACR Standards for Teleradiology.* Reston, Va.: American College of Radiology; 1994.
95. National Electrical Manufacturers Association. Digital imaging and communications (ACR-NEMA Standards Publication No. 300). Reston, Va.: ACR, 1994.
96. Di Matteo MR, Taranta A, Friedman HS, Prince LM. Predicting patient satisfaction from physicians' non verbal communication skills. *Med Care.* 1980;18: 376–387.
97. Johnson TM, Hardt EJ, Kleinman A. Cultural factors in the medical interview. In: Lipkin M, Putman SM, Lazare A, eds. *The Medical Interview.* New York: Springer-Verlag; 1995:153–177.

98. Becker MH. Patient adherence to prescribed therapies. *Med Care.* 1985;23: 539–555.
99. Wurmser L. *The Mask of Shame.* Baltimore: Johns Hopkins University Press; 1981.
100. Balint M. *The Doctor, His Patient and the Illness.* New York: International Universities Press; 1972.
101. Salmon P, May CR. Patients' influence on doctors' behavior: A case study of patient strategies in somatization. *Int J Psychiatry Med.* 1995;25:319–329.
102. Holm S. What is wrong with compliance? *J Med Ethics.* 1993;19:108–110.
103. Freidin RB, Lazerson AM. Terminating the physician-patient relationship in primary care. *JAMA.* 1979;241:819–822.
104. Lupton D. Perspectives on power, communication and the medical encounter: Implications for nursing theory and practice. *Nursing.* 1995;2:157–163.
105. Glenn ML. Separation anxiety: When the therapist leaves the patient. *Am J Psychother.* 1971;25:437–464.
106. Quill TE. Partnerships in patient care: A contractual approach. *Ann Intern Med.* 1983;98:228–234.
107. Bertakis KD. The communication of information from physician to patient: A method for increasing patient retention and satisfaction. *J Fam Pract.* 1977;5:217–222.
108. Fletcher SW, Fletcher RH. Patient's understanding of prescribed drugs. *J Community Health.* 1979;4:183–189.
109. Anonymous. Telemedicine: Fad or future? [editorial]. *Lancet.* 1995;345:73–74.
110. Perednia DA. Fear, loathing, dermatology, and telemedicine. *Arch Dermatol.* 1997;133:151–155.
111. Filberti D, Wallace D, Koteeswaran R, Neft D. A telemedicine transaction model. *Telemedicine Journal.* 1995;1:237–247.
111a. Advisory Committee on Telecommunications and Health Care. *Federal Communications Commission White Paper.* Oct. 15, 1996.
112. Uldal SB, Sund T, Stoermer J. Four years with teleradiology: A technical description. *Telemedicine Journal.* 1997;3:235–241.
113. Halliday BE, Bhattacharyya AK, Graham AR, et al. Diagnostic accuracy of an international static-imaging telepathology consultation service. *Hum Pathol.* 1997;28:17–21.
114. Becker-RL J, Specht CS, Jones R, Rueda PM, O'Leary TJ. Use of remote video microscopy (telepathology) as an adjunct to neurosurgical frozen section consultation. *Hum Pathol.* 1993;24:909–911.
115. Shimosato Y, Yagi Y, Yamagishi K, et al. Experience and present status of telepathology in the National Cancer Center Hospital, Tokyo. *Zentralbl Pathol.* 1992;138:413–417.
116. Eide TJ, Nordrum I, Stalsberg H. The validity of frozen section diagnosis based on video-microscopy. *Zentralbl Pathol.* 1992;138:405–407.
117. Weinstein RS, Bloom KJ, Rozek LS. Telepathology and the networking of pathology diagnostic services. *Arch Phys Med Rehabil.* 1987;111:646–652.

118. Weinstein RS, Bloom KJ, Krupinski FA, Rozek LS. Human performance studies of the video microscopy component of a dynamic telepathology system. *Zentralbl Pathol.* 1992;138:399–403.

119. Schiffer M. Legal aspects of telepathology. *Zentralbl Pathol.* 1992;138:393–394.

120. Burgiss SG, Julius CE, Watson HW, Haynes BK, Buonocore E, Smith GT. Telemedicine for dermatology care in rural patients. *Telemedicine Journal.* 1997;3:227–233.

121. Clark RA, Rietschel R.L. The cost of initiating appropriate therapy for skin diseases: A comparison of dermatologists and family physicians. *J Am Acad Dermatol.* 1983;9:787–796.

122. Kvedar JC, Edwards RA, Menn ER, et al. The substitution of digital images for dermatologic physical examination. *Arch Dermatol.* 1997;133:161–167.

123. Oakley AM, Astwood DR, Loane M, Duffill MB, Rademaker M, Wootton R. Diagnostic accuracy of teledermatology: Results of a preliminary study in New Zealand. *N Z Med J.* 1997;110:51–53.

124. Jones DH, Crichton C, Macdonaldd A, Potts S, Sime D, Toms J, McKinlay J, ed. Teledermatology in the highlands of Scotland. In: Wootton R, *Belfast: Institute of Telemedicine and Telecare;* 1995; 20–22.

125. Reponen J, Lahde S, Tervonen O, Ilkko E, Rissanen T, Suramo I. Low-cost digital teleradiology. *Eur J Radiol.* 1995;19:226–231.

126. Scott-WW J, Bluemke DA, Mysko WK, et al. Interpretation of emergency department radiographs by radiologists and emergency medicine physicians: Teleradiology workstation versus radiograph readings. *Radiology.* 1995;195:223–229.

127. Stormer J, Bolle SR, Sund T, Weller GE, Gitlin JN. ROC: Study of a teleradiology workstation versus film readings. *Acta Radiol.* 1996;38:176–180.

128. Goldberg MA, Rosenthal DI, Chew FS, Blickman JG, Miller SW, Mueller PR. A new high-resolution teleradiology system: Prospective study of diagnostic accuracy in 685 transmitted clinical cases. *Radiology.* 1993;186:429–434.

129. Halvorsen PA, Kristiansen IS. Radiology services for remote communities: Cost minimisation study of telemedicine. *Br Med J.* 1996;312:1333–1336.

130. Bailes JE, Poole RN, Hutchison MS, Maroon JC, Fukushima MD. Utilization and cost savings of a wide area computer network for neurosurgical consultation. *Telemedicine Journal.* 1997;3:135–140.

131. Baer L, Cukor P, Jenike MA, Leahy L, O'Laughlen J, Coyle JT. Pilot studies of telemedicine for patients with obsessive-compulsive disorder [see comments]. *Am J Psychiatry.* 1995;152:1383–1385.

132. Jerome L. Assessment by telemedicine [letter; comment]. *Hosp Community Psychiatry.* 1993;44:81.

133. Folsom JP. Clinical efficacy of telepsychiatry. *Telemedicine Journal.* 1995;1:187–188.

134. Bowersox JC, Shah A, Jensen J, Hill J, Cordts PR, Green PS. Vascular applications of telepresence surgery: Initial feasibility studies in swine. *J Vasc Surg.* 1996;23:281–287.

135. Bowersox JC. Telepresence surgery. *Br J Surg.* 1996;83:433–434.

136. Allen D, Bowersox J, Jones G. Telesurgery. *Telemedicine Today.* 1997;5(3):18–25.

137. Sackier JM. Phantoms and pixels, apparitions and apparatus: Image guided general surgery. *J Image Guid Surg.* 1995;1:75–79.

138. Cheriff AD, Schulam PG, Docimo SG, Moore RG, Kavoussi LR. Telesurgical consultation. *J Urol.* 1996;156:1391–1393.

139. Ball K, Perez J, Theslof G. Video conferencing in surgery: An evolving tool for education and preceptorships. *Telemedicine Journal.* 1995;1:297–302.

140. Finkelstein SM, Lindgren B, Prasad B, et al. Reliability and validity of spirometry measurements in a paperless home monitoring diary program for lung transplantation. *Heart Lung.* 1993;22:523–533.

141. Allen A, Hayes J. Patient satisfaction with teleoncology: A pilot study. *Telemedicine Journal.* 1995;1:41–46.

142. Hubble JP, Pahwa R, Michalek DK, Thomas C, Koller WC. Interactive video conferencing: A means of providing interim care to Parkinson's disease patients. *Mov Disord.* 1993;8:380–382.

143. Flowers CW, Baker RS, Khanna S, Ali B, et al. Teleophthalmology: Rationale, current issues, future directions. *Telemedicine Journal.* 1997;3:43–52.

144. Goldberg MA, Dwyer SJ. Telemammography: Implementation issues. *Telemedicine Journal.* 1995;1:215–226.

145. Celler BG, Lovell NH, Hesketh T, Ilsar ED, Earnshaw W, Betbeder ML. Remote home monitoring of health status of the elderly. *Medinfo.* 1995;8(pt 1):615–619.

146. Trippi JA, Kopp G, Lee KS, et al. The feasibility of dobutamine stress echocardiography in the emergency department with telemedicine interpretation. *J Am Soc Echocardiogr.* 1996;9:113–118.

147. Schanz SJ. Videotaping teleconsults: Pros and cons. *Telemedicine Today.* 1997;5:9.

148. Mossberg, W. Enjoying speedy link to the Internet after a slow start. *Wall Street Journal,* February 12, 1998.

149. Schanz SJ, Gordon EL. *1998 Compendium of Telemedicine Laws. Selected Statute Excerpts and Article Citations Relating to Telemedicine.* Raleigh, N.C.: Legamed Inc; 1998.

150. Alvarez A. Stung by U.S., Microsoft is forced to end isolationism. *New York Times,* December 21, 1997.

151. Bauch J. *Demosclerosis.* New York: Times Books, Random House; 1994.

152. Telemedicine prompts fears by state medical groups about big competitors. *Wall Street Journal.* January 17, 1996.

153. The Joint Working Group on Telemedicine. *(Legal Issues—Licensure and Telemedicine).* Telemedicine report to the Congress, January 31, 1997, Washington, D.C.: USGPO, 1997;27–51.

154. Schanz S, Gordon E. *Telemed Law: 1998 Compendium of Telemedicine Laws: Selected Statute Excerpts and Article Citations Relating to Telemedicine.* Raleigh, N.C.: Legamed; 1998.

155. Perednia DA, Allen A. Telemedicine technology and clinical applications [see comments]. *JAMA*. 1995; 273:483–488.
156. Booker, E. HMOs Rx: An Intranet. *Internet Week*, December 1, 1997, pp. 1–83.
157. Leitner PJ. Innovations create ripe climate for mainstream telemedicine adoption. *Telemedicine and Telehealth Networks*. 1998;4:31–34.
158. Health Care Financing Administration. *Health Care Financing Review*. Washington, D.C.: Author; 1996.
159. Allen A. Editor's note. *Telemedicine Today*. 1997;5(4):5.
160. Health Care Financing Administration and Bureau of Data Management and Strategy. Medicare persons served per HCFA region. Washington, D.C.: Author; 1996.
161. Organization for Economic Cooperation and Development. *OECD Health Data 1997*. Washington, D.C.: Author; 1997.
162. Peden EA, Freeland MS. A historical analysis of medical spending growth 1960–1993. *Health Affairs*. 1995;14:235–247.
163. Cowley L, et al. Magnetic resonnance imaging and marketing investment tensions between the forces of business and the practice of medicine. *Chest*. 1994;106:920–928.
164. Carey TS, et al. The outcomes and costs of care for for acute low back pain among patients seen by primary care practitioners, chiropractors and orthopedic surgeons. *N Engl J Med*. 1995;333:913–917.
165. Simon CJ, White WD, Gamliel S, Kletke PR. The provision of primary care: Does managed care make a difference? *Health Affairs*. 1997;16(6):89–98.
166. Hadley J, Mitchell JM. Effects of HMO market penetration on physicians' work effort and satisfaction. *Health Affairs*. 1997;16(6).
167. US Department of Health and Human Services. *States' assessment of health personnel shortages: Issues and concerns* (HRS-P-OD 90-6) Washington, D.C.: Author; 1990.
168. Stoddard J, Sekscenski E, Weiner J. The physician workforce. *Health Affairs*. 1998;17:252–257.
169. Rudd GL. Physician extender models reduce costs of telemedicine services. *Telemedicine and Telehealth Networks*. 1998;4:10–21.
170. Darkins A, Sibson L. The building of appropriateness. *The London Monitor*. 1996;3:82–86.
171. Boyle S, Darkins A. Health care markets: Abstract wisdom or practical nonsense. In: Harrison A, ed. *Health Care UK*. London: King's Fund Institute, 1994;63–71.
172. Boyle S, Darkins A. Purchasing specialist health care in London. *London Monitor*. 1994;1:40–44.
173. Kenney G, Rajan S, Soscia S. State spending for Medicare and Medicaid home care programs. *Health Affairs*. 1998;17:201–212.
174. Riverside Community Health Care, London. Community nursing activity data. Unpublished raw data.

175. Allen A. An Italian telephone mediated home monitorng service. *Telemedicine Today.* 1997;5:25.
176. Yatim L. An Israeli telenursing call center. *Telemedicine Today.* 1997;5:26.
177. Remington L. Interview. *Telemedicine Today.* 1995;3:22–23.
178. Doolittle G. A POTS-based tele-hospice project in Missouri. *Telemedicine Today.* 1997;5:18–19.
179. Goldberg A. Tele-home healthcare. *Telemedicine Today.* 1997;5:14–15.
180. Swett HA, Holaday L, Leffell D, et al. Telemedicine: Delivering medical expertise across the state and around the world. *Conn Med.* 1995;59:593–602.
181. Moscovice I, Casey M, Krein S. Expanding rural managed care: Enrollment patters and prospects. *Health Affairs.* 1998;17:173–179.
182. Navein J, Hagmann J, Ellis J. Telemedicine in support of peacekeeping operations overseas. *Telemedicine Journal.* 1997;3:207–214.
183. Zajtchuk J, Zajtchuk R. Strategy for medica readiness: Transition to a digital age. *Telemedicine Journal.* 1996;2:179–186.
184. Satava RM, Jones SB. Virtual reality and telemedicine: Exploring advanced concepts. *Telemedicine Journal.* 1996;2:195–200.
185. Whitten P, Allen A. Analysis of telemedicine from an organizational perspective. *Telemedicine Journal.* 1995;1:203–213.
186. Jones TL. Don't cross that line: Texas telemedicine law stirs up national debate. *Tex Med.* 1996;92:28–32.
187. Roberts EB, Fusfeld AR. Critical functions: Needed roles in the innovation process. In: Katz R, ed. *Career Issues in Human Resource Management.* Englewood Cliffs, N.J.: Prentice Hall; 1982:182–207.
188. Pelz DC. Creative tensions in the research and development climate. In: Katz R, ed. *Managing Professionals in Innovative Organizations.* Cambridge, Mass.: Ballinger, 1988;37–48.
189. Carey RG. Correlates of satisfaction in the priesthood. *Administrative Science Quarterly.* 1972;17:185–195.
190. White J, Ruh R. Effects of personal values on the relationship between participation and job attitudes. *Administrative Science Quarterly.* 1973;18:506–514.
191. Shapero A. Managing creative professionals. In: Katz R, ed. *Managing Professional in Innovative Organizations.* Cambridge, Mass.: Balinger; 1988; 215–222.
192. Swartz D. What's hot and what's not hot: Anticipating trends in technology. *Telemedicine Today.* 1997;5(5):28–32.
193. National Electrical Manufacturers Association. Digital imaging and communications (ACR-NEMA Standards Publication No. 300). Reston, Va.: ACR, 1989.
194. White K, Hoare J, eds. *Tidal Wave, New Technology, Medicine and the NHS.* London: King's Fund; 1992.
195. Sanderson, C. Evidence-based candidates for the audit and purchasing agenda. London: North Thames Regional Health Authority; 1996.
196. Nitzkin J, Zhu N, Marier R. Reliability of telemedicine examination. *Telemedicine Journal.* 3:1997;141–157.

197. Troyen A, Brennan, et al. The incidence of adverse events and negligence in hospitalised patients: Results of the Harvard Medical Practice Study. *N Engl J Med.* 1991;324:370–376.

198. Millenson M. First do no harm. In: Anonymous. *Demanding Medical Excellence.* London and Chicago: University of Chicago Press; 1997:63.

199. Cordner S. Australia's preventable deaths. *Lancet.* 1995;345:1562.

200. Ott JE, Bellaire J, Machotka P, Moon JB. Patient management by telephone by child health associates and pediatric house officers. *J Med Educ.* 1974;49: 596–600.

201. Lesar T, et al. Medication prescribing errors in a teaching hospital. *JAMA.* 1990;17:2329–2334.

202. Muir Gray JA. *Evidence-based healthcare: How to make health policy and management decisions.* London: Churchill Livingstone; 1997.

203. Canadian Task Force on the Periodic Health Examination. The periodic health examination. *Can Med Assoc J.* 1979;121:1193–1254.

204. Canadian Task Force on the Periodic Health Examination. The periodic health examination: 1984 update. *Can Med Assoc J.* 1984;130:1278–1285.

205. Canadian Task Force on the Periodic Health Examination. The periodic health examination: 1986 update. *Can Med Assoc J.* 1986;134:721–729.

206. Canadian Task Force on the Periodic Health Examination. The periodic health examination: 1988 update. *Can Med Assoc J.* 1988;138:617–626.

Glossary of Terms and Abbreviations

Adobe Acrobat Reader: A program created by Adobe, enabling the viewing of documents from multiple applications on a variety of platforms.

Analog: A continuous electrical impulse in waveform, which varies according to the nature of the information that is being sent. Typically, an analog signal is able to represent a physical characteristic such as the brightness and sharpness in visual images and loudness and pitch in sound.

Analog transmission: Data communication in which a physical dimension of the signal varies with time.

Application: A piece of software designed to meet a specific purpose.

Architecture: The layout and design that typifies the arrangement of an individual computer or a network of linked computers.

Asynchronous: An activity taking place independently of a set time signal.

Asynchronous communication: Electronic communication where there is an obligate delay between the sending and receipt of the data.

Asynchronous transfer mode (ATM): A type of switching system contained on an electronic data network that effectively bridges between packet and circuit switching.

Audio-speaker microphone unit: A sound communication device allowing a group of people to teleconference together from the same room. It is usually made up of a loudspeaker and several microphones that can interface with the videoconferencing unit or telephone system.

Bandwidth: An agreed measure of the capacity of a data channel to exchange information, providing a gauge of a network's capacity to carry data.

Baud: A measure of the rate at which digital data is transmitted over a data channel. Its units of quantification are usually described as bits per second, or bps;

consequently, a baud rate refers to the number of bits processed per second. In the case of a modem or fax machine, its baud rate denotes the highest rate at which it is capable of sending/receiving digital information.

Bit: The basic unit of information composed in binary code used by a computer to process data.

Bps: Bytes per second.

bps: Bits per second.

Broadband: A specific type of communication channel required by applications needing to transmit data containing a wide range of frequencies at high rates of data transfer, e.g., commercial broadcast TV and cable TV.

Broadcast: The directed transmission of information that makes it accessible to a wide and undifferentiated audience.

Browser: A software package for browsing the Internet, for example, Netscape Navigator, Mosaic, Chameleon, or Microsoft Internet Explorer.

Byte: Eight bits.

Cable modem: A modem that connects to to the cable television lines of cable companies to provide an incoming and outgoing Internet connection.

Cable providers: Commercial telecommunications companies that can provide data, telecommunications, entertainment, and Internet services via coaxial cable networks that are usually laid underground and available to home and business users.

Carrier: A government-regulated telecommunications company that is bound by set conditions governing the use of the network and how its services are charged for.

CD-ROM: Compact disk–read only memory, a data storage system for audio and data that is being challenged by DVD.

Client/server architecture: A network in which computer processing is distributed among numbers of individual personal computers (clients) and a more powerful central computer (server). Clients can share files and retrieve data stored on the server.

Clinical information system: A computer-based information system that can stand alone or networked to provide clinical data, including patient records, and clinical audit, and clinical risk management data. It may or may not be distinct from the administrative information system.

Cochrane Collaboration: An international network for evidence-based practice in health care.

Codec (code/decode):   A device for converting an analog signal into a digital signal for transmission and vice versa at the receiving end.

Collaborative software: Groupware such as the programs Microsoft Exchange and Lotus Notes.

Common gateway interface (CGI):   A UNIX application to allow the interchange of data between servers and Internet sites.

Compatibility: The ability for computer hardware and software to interchange and operate between different systems and still perform their function adequately.

Compression: The removal of redundant data that should not affect its later interpretation thereby facilitating the storage and transmission of data. Compression reduces the bandwidth required for high-speed data transfer. Compression is one factor in the time delay associated with in real-time videoconferencing.

Compression ratio: The ratio of the amount of data, in bits, of the original file/image to the amount in the compressed file/image.

Cookie: A fragment of software deposited on a computer after the user has visited a Web site. This enables the Web service provider to gather data and personal information about those who visit their site.

CT scanning: Computer tomographic scanning.

Data mining: The interrogation of databases or data warehouses to retrieve previously unknown information.

Data warehouse: A location, either virtual or physical, where data is stored.

Database: A software package for storing and retrieving data.

Dedicated line: A permanent connection between telephones and computers or videoconferencing units that does not require switching.

DICOM: Digital Image and Communication in Medicine, an industry and professionally agreed to standard for data communication between medical imaging devices that uses digital signals.

DICOM-RT: Digital Image and Communication in Medicine applied to radiation therapy.

Digital: The exchange of data using a constant stream of bits instead of the variable signal employed in analog communication.

Digitizing: The conversion of analog information (e.g., an x-ray film into digital form).

Direct digital imaging: The direct capture of x-rays and standard photographic images into digital form, without requiring the intermediary of film.

Domain name: The address of an Internet site (e.g., www.____.com or www.____.net).

DPI: Dots per inch, a measure of resolution for digital images.

ECG: Electrocardiogram.

E-commerce: Business transactions taking place electronically over the Internet.

EEG: Electroencephalogram, a recording of brain electrical activity from electrodes usually placed on the scalp.

Electronic data interchange (EDI):   The transmission of documents by means of electronic media using standard forms, messaging, and data elements.

E-mail: An electronic communication system between computers and computer systems allowing written messages to be sent between specified electronic addresses; includes the capacity to attach files.

Encryption: A data security technique in which digital information is recoded to make the bit stream unreadable to others who do not have the necessary system for restoring the data to its original form.

Enterprise resource planning: An integrated information technology solution that combines supply, logistical support, production, distribution, contract and order management, sales forecasting, finance, and human resource management.

Ethernet: A communications protocol used in networking that operates at 10Mbps.

Extranet: An extended intranet that uses Internet protocols and is accessible to people outside the organization's information system via the Internet.

Fiberoptics: Cables for data transmission that are composed of bundles of minute flexible glass rods. Light transmitted down these cables is used to transmit data, including audio and video signals.

Film digitizer: A piece of equipment to scan static images (e.g., x-rays) so that they can be stored or transmitted in digital form.

Filmless radiology: The use of direct digitizing so that x-ray images can be viewed, stored, and transmitted digitally on networks.

Firewall: A combination of hardware and software barriers to separate information networks to maintain security and prevent unauthorized acquisition of information, particularly important in health care to maintain the confidentiality of patient data. Or software that regulates access to a computer network from outside the immediate confines of the network.

Footprint: The area of the earth in which the transmission from a satellite can be received clearly.

Frame relay: A protocol for the transmission of data over networks whereby digital information is sent and received in the form of discrete packets.

Freeze-frame: A way of capturing and sending still images over standard telephone lines. Each signal image is transmitted and the picture updated approximately every 10 seconds.

Frequency: The rate of oscillation of an electromagnetic signal over time. This is usually measured in cycles per second, or Hertz.

Full duplex: A channel for data communication where transmission and receipt of information can occur simultaneously.

Full-motion video: A video signal that needs 6MHz in analog form and 45 Mbps in digital form to reproduce when transmitted.

GIF: A file extension definition to show that the file contains graphic images.

Groupware: Software that enables communication, collaboration, and coordination to take place between people who access an information system.

Half-duplex: A unidirectional data transmission link. Data can be sent and received but only one at a time.

Hardware: The physical component of the technology of computing on which a software program is installed and which undertakes the data processing. It is usually taken to mean the magnetic, optical, mechanical, and electrical components of a computer and its peripheral devices.

Hardwired: A permanent connection between technologies, as opposed to a removable or temporary connection.

HCFA: Health Care Financing Agency, the agency within the US Department of Health and Human Services that funds Medicaid and Medicare.

HDTV: High-definition television.

Health informatics: The application of computing and information science to manage the processes of data acquisition, information processing, and knowledge engineering in health care.

HIPAA: Health Insurance Portability and Accountability Act (US, 1996).

HIS: Hospital information system.

HMO: Health maintenance organization.

HTML (hypertext markup language):   With Java, it is the most common Internet programming language to create Web sites with their customary functionality.

HTTP (Hypertext transport protocol):   A means of connecting the various data elements drawn together on a Web site.

Image processing: The use of data refinement algorithms automatically or manually to improve the quality of digitally presented images for viewing.

Informatics: The application of computing and information science to manage the processes of data acquisition, information processing, and knowledge engineering.

Integrated circuit: Solid-state devices made from semiconductors that form the building blocks of the current "Information Age."

Integrated patient record: The concept of a patient record that can interface between health information systems so clinical information can be shared and duplication of data recording obviated.

Interface: A point at which discrete parts of computer hardware, software, and networks interconnect and across which data are transferred.

Internet: Currently the largest computer network in the world. It originated from bringing together computer networks in academic centers, government agencies, and commercial organizations throughout the world under the auspices of the US government. The Internet is in the process of being privatized, and there are plans for a new Internet to serve academic centers.

Intranet: A private network within an organization. Such a network is often protected from unauthorized access by a firewall.

IS Strategy (information systems strategy):   The process, usually formally recorded in a document, whereby priorities are identified and managed in an information system.

ISDN (Intergrated Service Digital Network):   A method of providing digital access to users on existing copper wire connections.

IT (information technology):   The combination of hardware and software used to manage and process information.

JAVA: A programming language used on the Internet, created by Sun Microsystems.

JPEG (Joint Photographic Experts Group):   A standard used for the compression of data to transfer digital images.

KM (knowledge management):   An ill-defined term that essentially refers to ways of maximizing an organization's use of data and information. This may involve creating, sharing, and leveraging the way data and information, both internal and external, are used in the organization to optimize its performance.

LAN (local area network):   A dedicated network allowing a defined group of organizations or individuals to communicate data in a closed system confined to a relatively small geographical area.

LATA (local access transport area, US):   Local areas for telephone provision created by the changes in the US telecommunications industry with the creation of seven regional telephone companies.

LDC: Long distance carrier.

Leased lines: Data communication lines that are rented from a communications carrier, so there are no individual call charges.

Legacy system: A software application, often a database that is obsolete and still in use.

Lossless: Data compression algorithm with a compression rate of 2:1, or below where there is no appreciable loss of quality when the image is reproduced.

Lossy: Data compression algorithms with higher compression rates, where there is appreciable loss of quality when the image is reproduced.

Mainframe: The central processing unit of a physically large computer system that usually receives input from a number of dedicated terminals linked directly to it. Ironically, current stand-alone PCs can be much more powerful than some older mainframes.

MAN: Metropolitan area network.

Medical informatics: The application of computing and information science to manage the processes of data acquisition, information processing, and knowledge engineering in medicine/health care.

Message switching: Dividing data to be transmitted into parts that are separately dispatched; the receiving site must combine these to re-create the original message.

Microprocessors: The basic building blocks, made up of complex electronic circuits, that provide a computer's processing power.

Microwave: High-frequency radiowaves, usually over 2 GHz, that can transmit data from point to point.

Minicomputer: An evolutionary step in the evolution of mainframes to the PC computer as computer use grew in the early 1970s.

Modem: Modulator/demodulator, a device to convert analog data to a digital format so that it can be sent over POTS (plain old telephone system). Reading the data requires another modem.

MPEG (Motion Picture Experts Group): A commonly agreed to compression standard for the exchange of digital video images.

MRI: Magnetic resonance imaging.

Multimedia: A combination of sound, graphics, animation, and video to present information or entertainment on a computer system.

Multiplexing: Linking together larger numbers of smaller, low-bandwidth data channels into a single high-bandwidth channel.

Narrowband: Under 1.544 Mbps data communication channel.

NASA: National Aeronautics and Space Administration (US).

NEMA: National Electrical Manufacturers Association (US).

Network: An arrangement of data nodes whereby users can exchange data.

NHS: National Health Service (UK).

Node: A point of entry for data exchange on a network.

On-line: The ability to communicate with others using a computer and a modem.

Operating system: The program that supports the internal functions of the computer and enables it to "know" the time and date and allocate memory.

Packet: A block of data that is transferred on a packet network.

Packet switching: A network transmission system involving the sending of data in discrete packets that can use different routes to arrive at their final destination if the network is busy with data traffic.

PACS: (Picture archiving and communications systems): Systems for the acquisition, transmission, sharing and viewing, storage, and retrieval of digital images (x-ray, CT, MRI) over a network.

PC (personal computer):   In the past this term was used to differentiate an IBM from a Macintosh computer. Now it refers to any personal computer, as distinct from a mainframe, laptop, or handheld device.

PDF: A file extension designating that it was created in Adobe Acrobat and therefore requires this program for subsequent viewing of the file contents.

Platform: A computer's operating system, hardware, and software in aggregate, used to indicate the functionality of the system in terms of what applications it can run.

Plug-in: A way of increasing the functionality of a Web browser's capability beyond its original design intention.

Pixel: The basic subunit of images presented on computer screens or CT and MRI monitors.

POTS: Plain old telephone system, the public service telephone system.

Process reengineering: A process of organizational change often associated with the use of information systems. It involves scrutiny of the core processes in the organization and devising a way to reassemble them more efficiently.

Program: The coded definition set that contains the instructions to enable a computer to perform a designated task.

Protocol: The languaging or messaging system one computer uses to speak with another.

PSN: Packet switched network.

PSTN: Public switched telephone network, the public telephone system.

Real-time: Data acquisition, processing, and presentation all occurring simultaneously in a system.

Repeater: A technological device used to amplify or regenerate communications signals on a network when it is sent over long distances. This is necessary because the signal is degraded over distance by the cable.

Resolution: A term used in the interpretation of images. Spatial resolution is the ability to differentiate defined structures present in an image. Contrast resolution is the ability to distinguish shades of gray in black-and-white images.

Routing: The process of assigning a path on a network for the transmission of data.

Satellite communication: The use of a device placed in earth orbit that functions as a retransmitter or repeater or electromagnetic signals to communicate data that can include video.

Search tool: A method of searching the Internet for data (e.g., Yahoo, Alta Vista).

Slow scan video: A transmission and receiving system for still video pictures over a narrow bandwidth connection.

Software: A term to describe the a program or set of programs that can run on a computer for a specific purpose.

SS7 (Signaling system 7): A development in the public telephone network that expands the functionality of the network. It does this by making call processing more efficient and enables the creation of new services that are being offered by communications carriers.

Store-and-forward: The transmission of still images or audiovisual clips from clinical consultations by a practitioner to a remote data storage device, from which they can be retrieved by a health care professional, usually a physician. This enables a practitioner to give his/her opinion on the consultation without the need for simultaneous availability of both clinicians. It makes teleconsultation more convenient and reduces the data costs because the bandwidth requirements for store-and-forward are lower than for real-time videoconsultation.

Switch: A mechanical or solid-state device that is used to open and close circuits, change operating parameters, or select paths or circuits on a space or time division. Switches are therefore used to route data communications on networks.

Switched line: A communication channel, such as the public telephone system, where the physical path decided at the time of dialing for the connection may vary with each use.

Switched network: A type of system in which every designated user has his/her own address, allowing the network to make a connection between any two users directly.

Synchronous transmission: A process for the transmission of bits of data at a fixed rate, with the transmitter and receiver systems both synchronized. This prevents interruption of the data transmission while it is in progress and improves the efficiency of communication.

Tariffs: The price structures used to regulate price for telecommunications in deregulated telecommunications markets. They are intended to ensure that telecommunications companies get fair return on capital and at the same time pass on savings to consumers.

T-carrier: Series of transmission systems using pulse code modulation technology at various channel capacities and bit rates to send digital information over telephone lines or other transmission media.

TCP/IP (Transmission control protocol/Internet protocol):   A communications protocol governing the exchange of data on the Internet.

Telecommunications: The use of wire, radio, optical, or other electromagnetic channels to transmit or receive signals that may carry audio, video, or data.

Teleconferencing: An interactive communication involving exchanges of voice, video, and data between people at two or more sites that is made possible by using telecommunications systems.

Teleconsultation: Health care consultations in which the participants are separated by geographical distance and also may be separated in time.

Telediagnosis: Making clinical diagnosis in health care on the basis of information relayed by a telehealth system.

Telehealth: See chapter 1.

Telematics: The use of computer-based information processing systems in telecommunications and the use of telecommunications systems for the transfer of data and programs between computer systems.

Telemedicine: See chapter 1.

Telementoring: The use of telecommunications media to provide individual guidance, instruction, or peer support.

Telemetry: The remote monitoring of information from patients using wire or radiotransmission, usually to establish diagnoses (e.g., telemetry to monitor EEG in epilepsy).

Telemonitoring: The use of telecommunications media to monitor the health status of patients at a distance.

Telepresence: The use of robotic and similar devices that make it possible for a person to perform a physical task (surgery, physical examination) at a distant site with the aid of a telecommunications system.

Throughput: The amount of data that a network can carry over a specified period of time.

Tie line: A leased or dedicated telephone circuit provided by a common carrier that links two sites without using the switched telephone network.

Trace route: A means of identifying the route taken by a computer to access a Web site.

Transmission speed: The rate at which data passes though a communications channel. It is measured in bits per second, or baud.

Transponder: A microwave repeater placed in a satellite for the purpose of receiving terrestrial signals, amplifying them, and then sending them back down to terrestrial receivers.

Trunk: A large-capacity channel that serves as the means for common carriers to exchange information between its users.

Twisted pair: The usual medium used in the public switched telephone network to make local connections. It is made up of insulated copper wires that are wrapped around one another to reduce interference. It is able to transmit voice, data, and low-quality interactive video.

Uplink: The path/link from a terrestrial station to a satellite for the transmission of data.

URL (uniform resource locator):   Usually a reference to a Web address site and the protocol needed to reach the site.

Validity: The degree of agreement between what is observed and what is real.

Videoconferencing: Real-time exchange of video images between two or more locations, usually two-way.

Virtual circuit: The appearance of an end-to-end circuit reproduced on a packet switched network.

Virtual domain: An Internet site appearing to be on its own dedicated server but in reality situated on a third party's server.

Virtual reality: A computer-generated simulation of visual, auditory, and other complex sensory stimuli.

Voice grade channel: A telephone circuit with the bandwidth necessary to transmit signals between 300 and 3,400 Hz.

Voice switching: An electronic switching device that opens and closes circuits in response to sound, usually verbal.

VRML (virtual reality markup language): A programming language, like HTML, to create virtual reality on the Internet.

WAN (wide area network): Data communications networks that provide long-haul connectivity between separate networks located in different geographic areas. By implication these are over a wide geographical area.

WATS (wide area telephone service): A telephone service with a measured bulk rate for long distance services.

Web server: Software placed on a Web site enabling it to respond to Web browsers.

WINSOCK: A Microsoft Windows link program to enable TCP/IP service interchange.

Workstation: A functional grouping of computer hardware and software (e.g., in telehealth—CD-ROM, monitor, camera) for individual uses such as teleconsultation.

World Wide Web: An Internet system for linking hypertext multimedia documents worldwide. It has now become a standard way for publishing and accessing information.

XML (Extensible Markup Language): A method allowing Web developers to define custom tags for marking and describing data. This enables data collaboration, information reuse, and interoperations to occur. This promises to do the same for data as HTML has done for graphics.

ZIP: A file extension designation to indicate that the file has been compressed to reduce its size for storage or transmission.

Index

Index

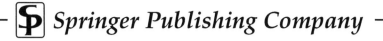

Springer Publishing Company

Distance Education in Nursing

Jeanne Novotny, PhD, RN, Editor

"The chapters in the book give a cross-section of ideas from various nursing programs across the country and give basic how-to-do information . . . The authors . . . share their expertise and the exemplary models of their programs." —**From the Introduction**

This is a comprehensive "how to" guide for designing, planning, and implementing a distance education program in a school of nursing. The emphasis is on web and internet based programs. Pioneers in this fast-emerging field share their experiences with readers -- both the ups and downs. These include nurses from the University of Colorado, University of Phoenix, the Frontier School of Midwifery and Vanderbilt University. The book is appropriate for nurse educators teaching undergraduate, graduate, advanced practice, and RN students.

Partial Contents: Distance Education Foundations, *J.M. Lewis* • Teaching a Web-Based Course: Lessons from the Front, *M.L. McHugh and R. Gibson* • Software Tools for Web Course Development, *R. Gibson and M.L. McHugh* • Clinical Applications of Electronic Learning Systems, *S.M. Moore and S.J. Kelley* • Assessing Distance Education Programs in Nursing, *K.L. Cobb and D.M. Billings* • Promoting Informatics in the Nursing Curriculum, *L.L. Travis* • Distance Graduate Education, *J.K. Magilvy and M.C. Smith* • Nurse Practitioner Education, *J.C. Novak and C.A. Corbett* • Distance Education at the Frontier School of Midwifery and Family Nursing, *S.E. Stone, E.K. Ernst, and S.D. Schaffer* • Supervision of RN Distance Learning Students, *C.J. Bess* • An International Education Model, *I. Lange, M. Urrutia, S. Jaimovich, and C. Campos* • The Future of Nursing Education: Marketability, Flexibility, and Innovation, *P.H. Walker*

2000   256pp   0-8261-1341-9   hardcover

536 Broadway, New York, NY 10012-3955 • (212) 431-4370 • Fax (212) 941-7842